Daniel Agusto

Harmonizing Your Craniosacral System

An Easy and Effective Self-Treatment

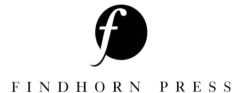

FINDHORN PRESS

Notice

The exercises described in this book are designed to enhance well-being and relaxation, and all are performed very gently. Craniosacral self-treatments support the comprehensive treatment of a craniosacral practitioner. They do not represent any substitute for orthodox medical and/or complementary medical diagnosis, or therapy. Assuming that you take care of your own health in a responsible way, these self-treatments are not supposed to be used for treating illnesses yourself. If you have health problems, you need to consult a medical doctor or an experienced alternative practitioner.

The responsibility for using these self-treatments lies with yourself. Author and publisher cannot be held liable for any damage to people, objects or property.

© Daniel Agustoni, 2003
English translation © Findhorn Press, 2008

First published in English by Findhorn Press, Scotland, 2008
Originally published in German by Kösel-Verlag GmbH & Co., Germany, 2004

ISBN 978 1 84409 117 1

A CIP catologue record for this title is available from the British Library.

Photos:
All exercises and models of the cranium by Tom Schneider; Graphics by Michael Hartmann and Susanne Noller – all © Sphinx-Craniosacral-Institut Basel, Switzerland
Models of the cranium pp. 11 and 103 © SOMSO

Translated by Sabine Weeke, edited by Jean Semrau
Cover design by Thierry Bogliolo
Interior design by Kösel Verlag, revised by Thierry Bogliolo

Printed and bound by WS Bookwell, Finland

Published by Findhorn Press, 305a, The Park, Findhorn, Forres IV36 3TE, Scotland, UK
tel +44 (0)1309 690582 • fax +44 (0)1309 690036 • eMail info@findhornpress.com

www.findhornpress.com

Contents

This book

is dedicated

to life,

love and

laughter

Foreword

by Dr. William Martin Allen

It is remarkable that the origin of Craniosacral Therapy began with an intuitive awareness by Dr. William Garner Sutherland that the cranial bones have mobility rather than being fixed and static. This realization by Sutherland initiated a lifetime of exploration that ultimately created a number of valuable approaches to Craniosacral Therapy.

Initially, the therapeutic model of Craniosacral Therapy involved a more mechanical approach to working with both the bones and membranes. Over time, the emphasis on working with the restriction of movement evolved into a more fluid and indirect approach by following the flow and direction of ease in the body, thus supporting more self-regulation and innate healing.

Today, the emphasis in Craniosacral Therapy has shifted from treating disease to accessing an individual's underlying blueprint of health, the inherent wisdom and source of all healing. Drawing upon his experience as a Craniosacral Therapist and teacher, Daniel Agustoni has provided a wide range of self-treatment protocols in a carefully-arranged order.

What I found in *Harmonizing Your Craniosacral System* to be particularly valuable are the following:

- The complex principles of Craniosacral Therapy have been described in a format that is easily accessible and thoroughly enjoyable to apply;
- The premise of the book promotes health by teaching individuals how to take responsibility for their own well-being through a series of Craniosacral self-treatment protocols;
- The text is both comprehensive and understandable, addressing the needs and interests of a wide spectrum of the population.

After multiple editions in German, *Harmonizing Your Craniosacral System* – both book and CD – are now available for worldwide distribution in English.

William Martin Allen, Ph.D, D.D.S.

Author's Preface

My interest in different kinds of relaxation techniques started about 20 years ago. Since 1987, following my trainings in traditional massage and biodynamic massage according to Gerda Boyesen, I have been interested in how people can treat themselves. In working with yourself, you deepen your body awareness and release tensions accumulated throughout the day more easily and more profoundly, even if you have only a few moments. Additionally, as an experienced craniosacral therapist I occasionally treat myself to a session of craniosacral therapy by another colleague.

Some of the exercises presented here I practice daily, either before getting up, during a break or before going to sleep. I have gotten used to those exercises; they have become part of my day. Depending on the situation, the environment and how my body feels, I intuitively choose those treatments that I feel are the right ones for me in the moment. These self-help exercises help me relax quickly and comfortably, also in my bathtub, in the warm water of a thermal bath or in the sauna.

Some self-treatments I have learned during my trainings, some I have modified. Many others I have developed, tested and optimized myself in the course of my years as a craniosacral practitioner. The concept and carefully chosen order of routines presented here originated in my own 13 years of experience in experimenting with them and in experiences with clients, patients and people who attended craniosacral workshops.

Starting in 1992 I introduced some of these practices into my massage courses as exercises in awareness and relaxation. For years now I have been teaching selected relaxation techniques to participants in craniosacral introduction evenings and basic craniosacral workshops. Practicing these in a group can enhance the effects even further.

Students of the craniosacral_flow® training learn the exercises presented here by sampling them for themselves, so that later in their own practice they are able to introduce to their clients those that are most effective for the individual. It is possible that craniosacral practitioners may slightly change these exercises in order to adapt them to the individual needs and abilities of the client.

The present exercises invite you to relax and feel well and at ease. By treating yourself you can spoil yourself in an effortless way. And you support your own good health: assisting the craniosacral system facilitates better self-regulation of the body.

Some of the instructions or sequences of the exercises are deliberately described like guided meditations. When you relax and become aware of yourself it is possible to get into contact with self-love, self-responsibility, boundary-setting, inner mindfulness. In deep relaxation further dimensions of being can open up.

My wish for and at the same time invitation to you is to let your body work with its inner rhythms and wisdom in these exercises. This corresponds to a basic principle by William G. Sutherland, originator of this method: "Let the liquids do the work!" Do not force yourself to anything. Touch yourself gently; give yourself plenty of space and time in all exercises – also in order to enjoy the relaxation.

If you do not feel well with or are not quite sure about some exercises, just leave them aside. You can of course turn to a craniosacral practitioner in order to experience the treatments and this possibly new feeling in your body with an adept companion.

I wish you much joy, equanimity and above all well-being and wonderful relaxation with these exercises.

Daniel Agustoni
Basel, Summer 2003

Introduction

Unhealthy stress and natural relaxation

Tension and relaxation are a natural principle, just like day and night, and the inner and the outer. Nowadays we have a huge range of stimuli flooding our senses, be it through radio, television, computer, mobile (cell) phone or internet.

In addition, we often experience increasing pressure and stress at work or in our private life. Much attention is focused on the "outer." Consequently fewer and fewer people can relax in a natural way and allow their body, mind and spirit the necessary rest. The autonomic nervous system of many people in the Western culture is set to a high degree on stress and therefore on activating the sympathetic nervous system. If the natural pendulum swing of tension and relaxation — or "inner" and "outer" — is disregarded for a period of time, sooner or later health and life quality will suffer. Permanent stress and possible consequences like back problems, chronic sleeping disorders or heart attack are quite common.

Also disastrous is the fact that many people — particularly those in helping professions — almost crucify themselves in that tension between inner calling and the constant excessive overload that makes them sick in the long run, and thus burnt out at some point (Burnout Syndrome).

Treating yourself

Since the demands we face will probably not diminish and possibly will even grow, we surely have to prioritize finding a new, more conscious way of being with ourselves and our stress.

For years I have been experiencing how people with many different mindsets have been able to relax within a few minutes through working with the craniosacral exercises. Treating yourself offers a healthy antidote to the stress of daily life.

The craniosacral exercises enhance and support:
- body awareness, deeper body sensation, increased awareness inside and out;
- relaxation through gentle touch instead of rough manipulation;
- sensitization of all senses, in particular the sense of touch;
- self-regulation, immune defense and regeneration of the body;
- growth processes, particularly in children and teenagers;
- inner peace.

The loosening-up exercises, self-massages, and awareness and palpation exercises are suitable for school children, teenagers and adults. They can also be used in guided groups – e.g., in school classes, sports and callisthenics groups or relaxation trainings.

The craniosacral exercises are suitable for:
- lay people who have already received craniosacral treatment and are free of pain;
- lay people with knowledge of massage and body therapies;
- people training to become craniosacral practitioners;
- craniosacral practitioners who want to offer and introduce their clients to exercises;
- physiotherapists, practitioners of other body therapies, alternative practitioners, midwifes and other professionals.

Engage in these craniosacral exercises with your unbiased openness, child-like wonder and great gentleness. There is nothing to achieve – the relaxation is simply waiting to be allowed in.

Observe which of the exercise routines in which format feel good to you and let the arising well-being and relaxation deepen. This means that you take responsibility for your own health. The exercises are there to support you in this.

Exercises in Part 1

Help us slow down and move more into our own center.

Exercises in Part 2

Relax the body and increase our awareness of our body.

Exercises in Part 3

Enhance deep relaxation; they relax the craniosacral system, in particular the mantle of our central nervous system and the flow of the cerebrospinal fluid (Liquor cerebrospinalis).

Only with some effort can we achieve relaxation, but we definitely cannot force it. Because relaxation is a natural principle (and an antidote to tension), body, mind and soul are only waiting for us to allow ourselves to let go and sink deeper into relaxing. In the end it happens by itself, and it deepens through meditative observation, through non-judgmental awareness, through not interfering, through allowing and surrender.

The Craniosacral System

The main focus of this book is the exercises for deepening awareness of and tuning into our body, and simple ways of treating the craniosacral system ourselves. I do not intend to give a comprehensive overview of the craniosacral system and craniosacral therapy here: you can find that in my book *Craniosacral Rhythm: A practical guide to a gentle form of bodywork therapy* (Elsevier, 2008) and in other technical literature; recommendations are given in the Appendix.

For some information on what treatment with a craniosacral practitioner can achieve and how it is performed, turn to page 130.

To help you visualise the exercises more fully, further illustrations and photographs of the craniosacral system, in particular of the cranial bone, may be found in Part 3, "Harmonizing the Craniosacral System" (with the respective exercises, pages 102 and 103).

The craniosacral system consists of:
- externally: the cranium (Cranium), the spine (Columna vertebralis) and the sacrum (Os sacrum) – therefore the name "craniosacral";
- internally: the meninges of the brain and spinal cord, which form the mantle of the central nervous system;
- the cerebrospinal fluid (Liquor cerebrospinalis).

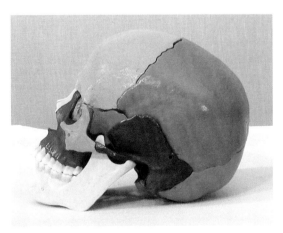

Cranial bones
sideways

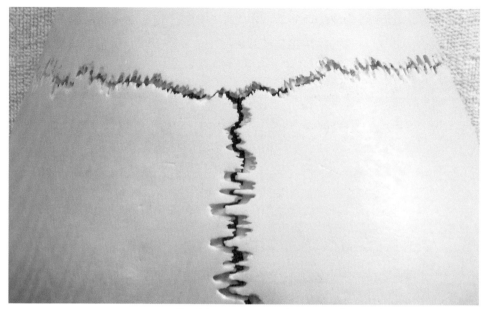

Cranial sutures: coronal suture and sagittal suture with bregma

Through directly or indirectly relaxing the craniosacral system, the cranial sutures, which connect the cranial bones with each other like joints, become more flexible and loose. At the same time the cranial bones carry gentle relaxation to the meninges of the brain and spinal cord (and further structures linked with them). Thus excessive tension of the meninges of the brain and the spinal cord is released and the fluctuation of the cerebrospinal fluid is improved. This aids the whole craniosacral system, the craniosacral rhythm and therefore the self-regulation and self-healing capabilities of the body.

Two examples:
- Relaxing the parietal bones will gently relieve tension in the large area of the meninges lying underneath and in the Falx cerebri, among other areas. The Falx cerebri is an inversion consisting of dura mater between the left and the right sides of the cerebrum; it forms the major part of the vertical plane of the intracranial membrane system of the cerebrum.
- Treating the temporal bones – in particular through the technique of "earpull" – relaxes the cerebellum (Tentorium cerebelli), which forms the horizontal plane of the intracranial membrane system of the cerebrum.

These relaxations support, for example:
- concentration and learning abilities;
- better blood circulation in the cerebrum;
- reduction/decrease of tension in the cranium and the area of the cervical vertebrae;
- the endocrine system and further functions of the body (see pages 16-17).

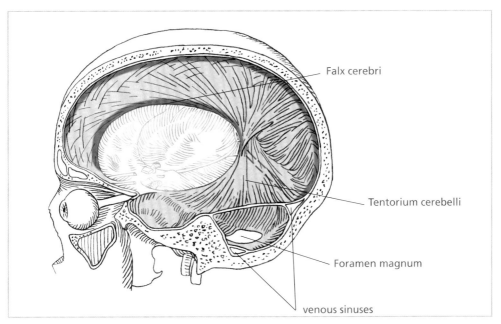

Falx cerebri

Tentorium cerebelli

Foramen magnum

venous sinuses

Falx cerebri, Tentorium cerebelli – side view

The spinal dura mater between occipital bone and sacrum

The meninges of the cranium continue after the great foramen magnum, underneath the base of the skull, as meninges of the spinal cord (Dura mater spinalis – separately: Dura mater, Arachnoidea, Pia mater) until they reach the coccyx (Os coccygis). This entire area is called spinal dura mater, or dural tube. The craniosacral rhythm is transmitted, among other routes, via the spinal dura mater from the occipital bone down to the sacrum where it can also be palpated – i.e., felt – if the tissue is free of restrictions.

Harmonizing Your Craniosacral System

The spinal dura mater is attached:

- to the foramen magnum of the occipital bone;
- inside the spinal cord in the area of the second and third cervical (C2/3);
- in the upper area of the sacrum (S2).

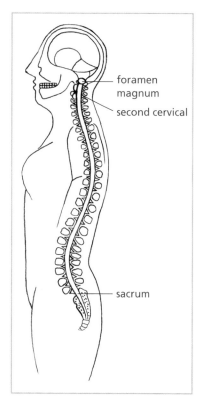

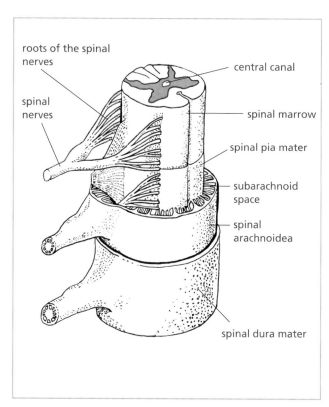

Spinal dura mater, intracranial membranes with attachment points

Spinal dura mater, spinal arachnoidea, exit of spinal nerves, spinal marrow

The cerebrospinal fluid (Liquor cerebrospinalis)

The cerebrospinal fluid is generated from the arterial blood. It is produced in the network of the Plexus choroideus on the walls of our ventricles of the brain (cerebric chambers/ventricles). Fluids are essential carriers and repositories of energy and information. The founder of osteopathy, Andrew T. Still, has said, "The cerebrospinal fluid is the highest known element in the body," and "The cerebrospinal fluid is like liquid light."

In the area of the interbrain/3rd ventricle, the cerebrospinal fluid is likely influenced by the excitation of both parts of the thalamus that control the frequency and the activity of the brain. Recent research has shown that the cerebrospinal fluid carries, for example, hormonal information from the pituitary gland (hypophysis) and the pineal gland (epiphysis) and distributes this throughout the entire central nervous system. Here we can also assume interactive neurological interactions, which are influenced by information from all levels of our being (body as well as mind and soul).

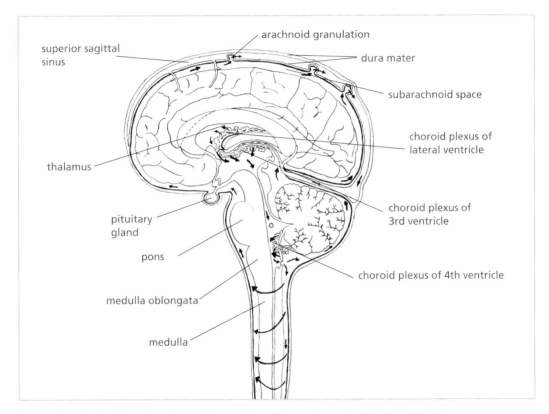

Production, distribution, allocation and resorption of the cerebrospinal fluid in the brain

The cerebrospinal fluid has important functions:

- *Protection:* the cerebrospinal fluid protects our brain and medulla. It has a specific weight similar to that of our brain, which by itself weighs about 1350 grams. But through the cerebrospinal fluid and the envelope of the meninges and the intracranial pressure, an apparent weight of only about 50 grams is generated.

- *Nourishment:* With its rich composition – among others, glucose, various proteins and substances dissolved in salt like sodium, calcium, magnesium, potassium – the cerebrospinal fluid assists in the brain's functions. Also detected are endorphins and neurotransmitters.

- *Cleansing and purification:* About four to seven times in 24 hours, approximately 110 to 170 ml of fluid in the entire craniosacral system is being renewed. The fluctuation and different pressure of the cerebrospinal fluid – about 500 to 700 ml are produced on a daily basis – take care of disposing of old brain and medulla cells via the venous blood and the lymphatic system.

- *Potential for transmitting and acting for the central nervous system:* The central nervous system is supported by metallic ions such as sodium, potassium and calcium in the cerebrospinal fluid.

The cerebrospinal fluid in particular is reabsorbed into the sagittal sinus (Sinus durae matris) in the area of the skullcap. With increasing pressure of the fluid, it is diverted via the arachnoid granulation (Granulationes arachnoidales) into the venous system. Along the spinal dura mater the fluid can spread via nerve exit points into the body where is it collected by the lymph system and removed.

The craniosacral system and its relationship to other body systems

The craniosacral system and other body systems – circulation (arterial and venous blood supply), nervous system, endocrine system (hormonal system), lymph system, respiratory system, musculoskeletal system (muscles, connective tissue, fascias, ligaments, tendons, joints) – are closely connected and influence each other.

The relaxation of the craniosacral system and the successively more pronounced movements of the craniosacral rhythm support these body systems individually and harmonize them as a whole.

The following body systems will be directly or indirectly affected and balanced:

- Entry and exit points of cranial nerves obtain more space to exercise their function more fully. This has a positive effect on the processing of all motor and sensory impulses.

- The balance of the autonomic nervous system is enhanced. This also supports the reduction of stress and general processing of outer impulses.

- The whole body profits from relaxing the muscles and the connective tissue. These cover the craniosacral system in part peripherally, in part directly. Surprisingly, many muscle insertions and ligaments are connected with bones of the craniosacral system. Too much tension in the muscles and the connective tissue impacts the craniosacral system. A hardened shoulder girdle, for example, will constrict the upper thoracic vertebrae, the cervical vertebrae and the transition to the cranium, which can affect the posture and cause headaches. The tension of the entire connective tissue also determines whether and how the craniosacral rhythm is perceptible on the whole body.

- Circulation: Also vitally important is a well-functioning arterial and venous blood supply, to prevent cerebral infarcts and heart attacks, for example.

- The lymph flow contributes to the detoxification and purification of the body.

- The endocrine system contributes to managing emotional reactions, sleep, hormonal secretion, body temperature, water balance, blood pressure and hunger. Thanks to intensive research, more and more connections are being discovered. The endocrine system's vital functions for the human being and its influence on the physical, mental and soul level are undisputed. The development of the human body and its well-being depend on a well-functioning and well-managed endocrine system. A free craniosacral rhythm drains and stimulates all areas of the brain and the entire body in a subtle way from the inside out.

More about the craniosacral rhythm in Part 3, pages 67-72.

Distinction between craniosacral therapy and craniosacral self-treatment

Craniosacral self-treatments support treatments by professional craniosacral practitioners. What such a treatment can look like and which effect it can have are briefly summarized at the end of this book (see page 130).

Craniosacral self-treatments form a part of the comprehensive training in craniosacral_flow®, the training concept I have developed. Many clients of craniosacral therapy are surprised what a pleasurable and deep effect such gentle bodywork can have. In the course of about 6 to 12 sessions most clients develop an expanded body awareness. In between those professional craniosacral treatments this awareness can be deepened through practicing the exercises given in this book.

Important guidelines for treating yourself

Before we start with the practical part of the book, I would like to share some basic advice to assist with the respective exercises. I have divided the treatments according to themes for better orientation. You will find the following three sections:

Loosening-up exercises and self-massages (Part 1)

These comprise general exercises for loosening up and "arriving at yourself" more fully. If you have no or little experience with relaxation techniques I recommend starting with this section of exercises, whereby you relax the craniosacral system in a predominantly indirect way. Most of these exercises you perform either standing or sitting. They constitute an optimal preparation for all self-treatments in Parts 2 and 3.

Awareness and tuning-in exercises (Part 2)

These are simple opportunities to relax the body with minimal technique and gentle touch. Among other things they help to relax the craniosacral system indirectly as well as directly. Primarily performed lying down or sitting, these awareness and tuning-in exercises invite you to raise the awareness around your body. They constitute optimal preparation exercises for the self-treatments in Part 3.

Harmonizing the craniosacral system (Part 3)

This section explains self-palpation and self-treatments for relaxing the craniosacral system. They bring you partly indirectly but mostly directly into contact with the craniosacral system. You conduct these exercises without forcing anything, touching yourself in a very gentle, careful way. They are mostly performed lying down or sitting. In order to be able to start from a basically relaxed space, I recommend using some of the self-treatments in Parts 1 and 2 as preparation. Three examples of self-treatment combinations are listed on pages 139–140.

How to perform the exercises

All self-treatments presented here are performed gently and slowly. They will achieve well-being and relaxation if you allow yourself and your respective body part much time, being mindful of and perhaps marvelling about the sensations that might reveal themselves in the moment. Times given are therefore relative and negligible. You decide from within – intuitively – whether you spend only 30 seconds or 10 minutes on one treatment (see also pages 26–27).

It is beneficial to start off in a calm space within yourself, with no pressure to achieve anything. Expectations of success would only create unnecessary stress and decrease the effect of the exercises.

If you find an exercise uncomfortable, just leave it aside.

The slow and gentle touches of torso, neck and head are as light as the wing beat of a butterfly

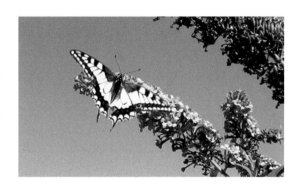

Do not compromise yourself and your craniosacral system in any way by a fast or forced approach. The exercises or hand positions themselves are not the goal, they are the path. On this path you get to know oases of well-being, relaxation and deep regeneration; more and more you will experience the unity of body, mind and soul.

If you have already treated yourself to an individual craniosacral session, you know how wonderful it is to be allowed to just lie down for about an hour and stop doing anything actively. The sensitization that you have experienced during such sessions will also help you to experience the quality and gentleness of these exercises for treating yourself.

You perform these treatments without effort and by choice, partly standing, mostly sitting or lying down. Some of the relaxation exercises that can be performed in a sitting or lying position can also be carried out in warm water – for example, in the bathtub. Weightlessness and the soft warm element of water facilitate and encourage the process of letting go.

The routines may be carried out with joy and lightness. Just enjoy the moments in which you need to do little or nothing. Every effort can be dropped. Maybe you will enter into something like a "timeless time." You can direct your effortless attention to the increasing feeling of well-being. Notice occasionally those parts of your body that feel most pleasurable. Thus the path is cleared for natural relaxation, which can intensify and expand into deep relaxation. Relaxation is our birthright!

During the exercises occasionally close your eyes and notice how this feels. The activity or technique is not what counts; rather it is your mindfulness and perception of the increasing well-being, the relaxed breathing and the sensation of letting go more and more.

Treating yourself leads to more self-awareness and self-love. It teaches us to differentiate between pressure, touch and "listening," and enhances awareness through touch. And this is particularly beneficial for the exercises in Part 2 and 3.

Human predispositions and abilities to sense and perceive nuances with all our senses are immense. That is why it is less of a question whether we can, for example, palpate subtle tissues or listen to slow body rhythms at all. What is crucial is that we begin to trust our hands and our bodily sensations. We can rediscover that our hands and our receiving presence are a sensitive instrument that is tuned and trained with every practice of palpating.

You can notice the relaxation in the tissue underneath your hands becoming:

- more spacious;
- softer;
- warmer;
- fuller.

When you softly feel and relax body structures, the so-called "therapeutic pulse" (see also page 74) can become noticeable at the spot touched, through:

- release of heat or coldness;
- twitching of muscles, discharges;
- strong throbbing or pulsing.

These signs show that the tissue with its "cell memory" starts to relax. At the same time you might perceive:

- hardening or softening of the tissue;
- heaviness or lightness;
- a streaming or flowing of energy/warmth in the body;
- pictures, colours or possibly a fragrance;
- a memory coming up.

Observe all this and continue to keep your attention where your hands are touching your body.

How do you sense the tissue after feeling the therapeutic pulse? What has changed? Has the local relaxation shifted anything in your body and/or your well-being?

Effects of the self-treatments

Relaxing strengthens our autonomic nervous system with its parasympathetic parts and thus supports our self-regulation and regeneration from the inside. A nervous system that regulates itself to a high degree oscillates quite fast between tension and relaxation, depending on the situation. This allows us to recover deeply and quickly in short breaks. The regenerating, reviving force with which we reconnect in relaxation is a regulating natural principle striving for wholeness and perfection. In combination, relaxation and self-regulation act as a fountain of youth: they boost the flow of energy, the life force, our immune system and our inner balance.

Often one perceives, for example, how the breathing changes, how shoulders and lower jaw drop or that peristalsis (stomach-bowel sounds) starts up. This shows that the person is releasing tension: the body starts to relax, the autonomic nervous system regulates itself and gets the chance to balance itself from the inside.

The visible and perceptible change in the individual is being confirmed again and again by experts as much as by laypeople. Many report that they can relax more deeply than they have been able to do for a long time, or that afterwards they feel as if they had had a good night's rest. They also experience qualities like clarity, equanimity, contentment, presence and focus. The "inner" as well as the "outer" is being perceived more acutely with all senses. Others feel more vital, more alive or report experiencing more contrast and colour in their vision – all via an enhanced, more sophisticated perception.

Many of the following self-treatment and awareness exercises constitute a subtle body awareness training at the same time. They invite you to treat yourself and your body with love, to trust it and listen to its inner wisdom with its varying slow rhythms.

It is of particular value to consciously feel the relaxation and perceive its beneficial effect afterwards. Thereby the new body feeling can deepen and anchor itself. Consciously observing the difference before and after also means that our brain notices this and stores the new body feeling. The more you connect with resourced body parts and rest in the holistic body awareness (supported by the exercises in this book), the more effective positive changes can establish themselves as they are thereby also anchored neurologically and in the subconscious mind. The mental level as well as the autonomic nervous system (by including the breathing) will also register and memorize the changes. Relaxation harmonizes the craniosacral system and supports all body systems in their functions (see pages 16–17).

All exercises in this book have effects on a large scale.

They enhance:
- the ability to learn and concentrate;
- sensors, motor function and balance;
- digestion, purification/detoxifying.

They support:
- free breathing;
- posture, back, the entire musculoskeletal system;
- harmonization of the whole body, the emotions and the soul.

They assist:
- in relaxation;
- in going to sleep;
- before and after stressful situations like an exam, a visit to the dentist, etc.;
- in gaining relaxation even from short breaks well spent.

These are only a few examples out of a variety of possible modes of action as the self-treatments can affect individual people differently. You will find some further examples with every exercise.

When you should not treat yourself

On no account should these self-treatment exercises be used as self-the-rapy when ill or after accidents, shock or trauma, without proper therapeutic monitoring. This is because in these cases the self-regulation ability of the body is often impaired to such an extent that help from outside is needed – e.g., from a medical practitioner, an alternative practitioner, a craniosacral expert or a trauma therapist. Also, when, while treating yourself strong feelings surface that swamp you, professional support is beneficial or indeed vital. You will find resources for this in the Appendix of the book.

- Contraindications for treating yourself in the head region – see page 123.
- Contraindications for stillpoints on the head – see page 86.

About the order of the self-treatment exercises

Becoming slow, smooth and gentle

I recommend beginning with one or two exercises from Part 1, "Loosening-up exercises and self-massages," continuing with some "Awareness and tuning-in exercises" from Part 2, and only then starting with exercises from Part 3, "Harmonizing the Craniosacral System."

If you are already very relaxed or familiar with gentle body therapy, you can start anywhere – i.e., perform the exercises separately, create your individual treatment programme in any order or follow the suggested order.

Three examples of combinations of self-treatments are listed on pages 139–140.

Important considerations before starting

The more you relax in treating yourself and allow space for yourself and your body, the wiser it is to create optimal conditions right from the start.

If you have done this a few times – maybe with a brief preparation ritual, looking forward to allowing yourself the space to relax soon – you will before long get into a habit of preparing yourself adequately. Your body will thus settle into well-being and relaxation more easily.

The following recommendations have proved to be of value:

Quiet and secure space

Always perform the exercises in a safe space. Make sure the surroundings are as quiet, safe and comfortable as possible, so that you are able to relax trustingly and without disturbances.

Fresh air

Before you start, air the room briefly but thoroughly in order to fill the space with fresh oxygen. Stuffy air can make you sleepy.

Room temperature

Depending on the season it might be advisable to slightly alter the room temperature. Most people find 20 to 24°C (68 to 75°F) comfortable when lying down.

Atmosphere in the room

Perhaps you would like to light a beautiful candle, freshen the room with subtle essential oils or support the exercises with appropriate music. You will find some music suggestions for the treatment and relaxation exercises in the Appendix.

If possible, decrease the volume of the answer phone, take your watch off or cover the clock, divert your mobile phone to voicemail or switch it off – even the noise of the vibration function can be disturbing.

Loose clothing

Make sure you wear comfortable clothing so as not to restrict the free flow of your breath. You should loosen or take off tight shirts, trousers, belts, watches, and jewelery. You do not need jogging trousers or sports dress; however, if you have them you can certainly wear them. Generally, though, ordinary clothes that do not constrict you are fine.

Warm blanket, pullover

It is advisable to have at hand a blanket or something warm to slip over yourself, in case your blood pressure drops during relaxation and/or you want to warm yourself up a bit. If you often suffer from cold feet, put on warm socks before you start the exercise.

Practice tips for the exercises

- First take a few deep breaths to enlarge your respiratory volume.
- Then continue breathing in a relaxed way; stay in the flow of breathing.
- Drop your lower jaw slightly.
- At times close your eyes. Thus your attention formerly absorbed by the sense of seeing is available to the other senses.

If some exercises are difficult to perform or do not feel comfortable for you, just leave them out.

Exercises in standing position
The feet are parallel to each other, at about shoulder width. Always stay relaxed in knees, hips and pelvis, so that you are well grounded.

Exercises in sitting position
You sit grounded and feel your feet, legs, pelvis, ischium and sacrum.

Use a suitable seat, perhaps with cushion or a soft blanket, where you can sit comfortably and where you can also adapt the height of the seat. A stable stool is recommended. If you have a chair with backrest, try out whether you want to lean against it or slightly move forward in order to have your back free. Make sure that the base on which you are sitting does not pinch off the underside of your thighs. If this should be the case, just move further forward towards the edge of the chair.

If you treat yourself in a sitting position, with elbows placed on the table, you need to be sure that you sit low enough or that the table is high enough. It is important that you do not sit bent over but as straight and relaxed as possible. A folded blanket under the elbows can sometimes be helpful.

Exercises in a lying position
Be sure you have a soft, comfortable base of support. If there is no bed or smooth massage table close by, you can use the floor: a soft bedspread or yoga mat, a futon, a plastic mat (a simple camping mat, sleeping pad, gymnastic mat or rubber foam covered with a sheet) or an air mattress.

Cushion or head support: When lying on the back or the side, rest your head on a comfortable cushion or folded blanket, at a convenient level.

Most self-help exercises in a lying position are performed when lying on your back.

To relieve the back and the body, roll up a blanket and place that roll underneath your knees. Or place one or more blankets under your knees or legs in order to rest them slightly higher. At times feel from head to toe where and how your body touches the base of support.

Posture easy on the back

When lying down as much as when sitting up, always maintain a posture that is easy on the back.

To lie down

When sitting, roll yourself sideways along one side of your body, down onto the table or other surface.

To get up

Move yourself to a lateral position and sit up slowly. This means you roll your body sideways, slowly upwards, until you sit.

Give yourself time so that balance and blood circulation can get used to the change, and so that you may become aware of the new body sensations in sitting and later in walking.

The time factor

Each self-treatment comes with a recommendation of approximately how long it takes. This timing is not compulsory; please adapt the timing to your inner needs. While you are becoming familiar with the body parts and exercises, and your awareness for your perception deepens, performing the exercises can take a bit longer. The more familiar the exercises and the more you perceive, the more intuitively you will use them; the aspect of time becomes less important.

In case you have to move into the ordinary time level straight after the relaxation – e.g., for an important appointment or in order to reach public transport in time – I recommend setting an alarm. An alarm clock that does not tick at all or is hardly audible helps you not to be reminded of the time prematurely but allows you to remain in the "timeless time" as long as possible.

Allow sufficient time after the self-treatments

Tracing

At the end of the exercises allow yourself an additional 5 minutes or more for tracing or tracking the sensation, without doing anything. These are valuable moments of stillness which can deepen the experience. In addition they may help you to relax more quickly and easily the next time because body, mind and soul will remember this natural state. Consciously perceiving differences and changes (before–after) also helps to anchor the experience of relaxation more fully.

After every deep relaxation allow yourself enough time to trustingly adapt to the reality of everyday life again.

Energizing yourself – Becoming active again in everyday life

I recommend performing the change from relaxation to activity with sensitivity. When you are relaxed and start becoming active again, shield yourself sufficiently against hectic everyday life. You should also be able to fully respond to your environment in case you happen to be on the road afterwards.

Deeper and somewhat faster breathing gives you more oxygen and thus more power and alertness. The loosening-up exercises in Part 1 can be energizing when they are performed a bit faster.

1 Loosening-up exercises and self-massages

General relaxation exercises

In order to experience as much joy and relaxation as possible with the following loosening-up exercises and self-massages, I recommend reading the chapters "Introduction" (pages 8–10) and "Important guidelines for treating yourself" (pages 18-27). The information contained in these chapters is valuable and should be taken into account with all of the following exercises.

Most of the self-help exercises in Part 1 can be performed standing; some can be performed sitting as well as lying down.

Shake, loosen, stretch and straighten the body

Cats, dogs and other animals give us an example on a daily basis: with pleasure they loll and stretch several times a day. It seems that we can learn a lot from animals, in particular from our pets; instinctively they do what is good for them.

Once you have gotten over any initial reluctance around the exercises, your condition can change and bring out much joy and power, including euphoric episodes of happiness. Combined with strong breathing in and breathing out, the loosening-up exercises also have a vitalizing effect.

All movements in the exercises are designed to make you feel good!

The following loosening-up exercises promote:
- relaxed leg and pelvic muscles in order to be grounded, mobile and flexible;
- a loose, strong pelvic floor;
- free, comfortably-toned hip and buttock muscles;
- entire body posture and statics;
- the flexibility of sacrum, pelvis, spine;
- the whole torso, shoulder and neck area up to the base of the skull;
- the diaphragm, respiration and the craniosacral system.

Shaking and loosening the body   ca. 2 min.

standing, possibly sitting

Performing the exercise

1. Shake out your arms and hands slowly and languorously. Your shoulders, elbows, wrists and hands are very loose and flexible, including all fingers. You can release to the outside all tension in these areas by shaking it out tenderly through your hands and fingers. In doing so, consciously breathe out the tension.

   When you are standing you can move your weight onto one leg and lightly shake out the relieved leg as well as the foot. Then change sides and casually shake out the other leg, with loose knee and ankle joints, as well as foot and toes. When sitting, you can shake out the feet lightly, one at a time.

2. Grounded through the feet, smooth seesaw movements originating in the knees and the hips start to loosen up the pelvis, climbing up the whole torso and supporting the shaking and loosening in the area of the shoulders and the neck up to the arms, hands and fingers. After some voluntary movements they can become independent again – your body can perform the movements while your breath flows. Loosen your lower jaw while you observe and relax.

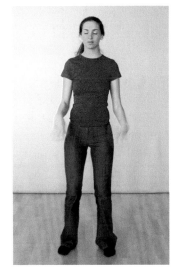

Shaking and loosening
the body

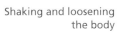

Muscle tapping, joggling and vibrating ca. 2 min.

standing, sitting, possibly lying down

Through long periods of sitting and stress, the muscles, tendons and ligaments of pelvis and thighs are often constricted, shortened and/or hard.

Performing the exercise

With the help of your arms, wrists and hands you loosen all your thigh and pelvic muscles through tapping, joggling and vibrating. In preparation, actively loosen up your wrists, shoulder and elbow joints by lightly shaking them out. To be on the safe side, do not use this exercise if you are afflicted with complaints like sciatic pain, lumbago or problematic varicose veins.

1. *Tap the muscles alternately*:
   - with open, slightly curved hands and supple wrists, or
   - with closed hands – i.e., formed into cushy fists.

   Make sure that your wrists are flexible and the palms or fists swing easily and loosely with the tapping movements of the mobile forearms.

   Tap rhythmically and relatively fast with your palms or loose fists:
   - the muscles of your thigh, the front as well as the back;
   - the lateral muscles of the pelvis;
   - around the major trochanter, very lightly, with the palms;
   - all pelvic muscles, in particular in places where you can feel many muscles;
   - sideways along the sacrum, then lightly on the sacrum;

You avoid the joints completely, or loosen or vibrate them only very lightly, with open palms (see photos).

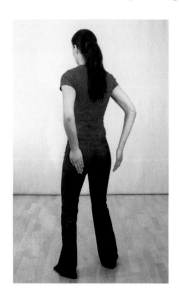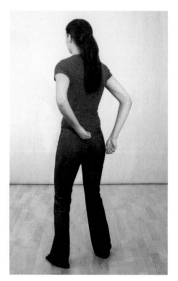

Light tapping of buttocks and sacrum

Left: with open palms
Right: with loose fists

2. You joggle your body on the same places that you have tapped before. For this your open palms touch as much skin and muscle surface as possible. Without sliding across the skin, joggle the structure underneath your hands to and fro rhythmically and relatively fast. Pay attention to the proper motion of the muscles and join in with their rhythm while joggling.

3. You vibrate in a similar way to the joggling, just a bit lighter. Here you do not move the muscles rhythmically to and fro, but vibrate the structure lightly on the surface. Increase the intensity of touch into the depth of the tissue, thus vibrating and loosening structures deeper within.

Stretching and straightening the body ca. 2 min. or longer

standing, sitting, lying down

Performing the exercise

You do not overextend but are connected with the light, vital positive tension in the body that you feel when gently stretching and straightening. With slow, feel-good exercises like lolling, stretching, straightening as well as yawning, sighing, feeling and breathing tension out, you express the tightness that you have experienced and let go of it with pleasure. The luxurious stretch and straightening movements can become increasingly flowing and can expand across the whole body. The entire torso and all extremities can be included. While doing this, every now and again breathe vigorously in and out.

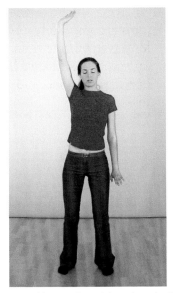 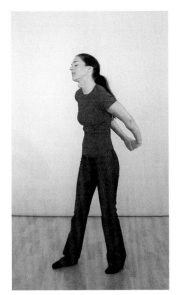 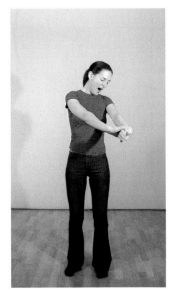

Stretching and straightening the body comfortably

Yawning

Lift and drop your lower jaw a few times and allow yourself to yawn strongly and loudly. Breathe out all tension and with every inbreath collect fresh air and power!

Tapping the thymus gland   ca. 1 min.

standing, sitting, lying down

The thymus gland is situated under the upper half of the breastbone (sternum). It is a primary organ of the lymphatic system, producing T-lymphocytes, and is of major importance for our immune system, the growth of the body and the metabolism of the bones.

Thousands of years ago, the Greeks knew that the thymus gland influences the life energy of the body. The Greek word "thymos" means "life force, life, soul, mind." In times of illness and stress the thymus gland reacts by decreasing in size. In times of harmony, balance of body, mind and soul, and when experiencing love, joy, trust, faith, confidence, the thymus gland increases in size. As a link between mind and body it seems to react to beautiful words and music by expanding.

Performing the exercise

Soft tapping on the breastbone stimulates the thymus gland and supports it in its function. While doing this let your lower jaw drop and your breath flow.

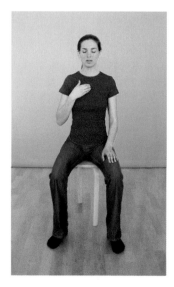

Tapping the thymus gland

Self-massages

Like all exercises in this book, the self-massages are to be performed calmly, without strenuous concentration, and so that they feel good. Let the breath flow freely and occasionally close your eyes while massaging yourself, in order to sense more clearly how it feels.

Begin slowly and without much pressure. Thus you are able to increase speed and pressure slightly while observing it at the same time. This is recommended so that you do not lose attention and your body does not produce unnecessary stress hormones because of pressure that is too rapid or too great. Massage yourself with love. Pause occasionally and touch the massaged area – listening, without actively doing anything.

Massaging ourselves is a good way of learning to distinguish between varying soft intensities of pressure and to occasionally touch for the purpose of listening only. This is also helpful for the self-treatments in Parts 2 and 3.

Foot massage   ca. 2 – 10 min.

sitting; possibly lying down, depending on the mobility
of the lower torso and hip area

Indulge yourself frequently – preferably on a daily basis – with an enjoyable foot massage during breaks or before you start off into the day. A natural massage oil like almond, arnica or jojoba oil is beneficial but not a prerequisite.

This self-massage promotes:
- flexible feet and ankles;
- our gait and whole posture;
- the prevention of dysfunctions that can travel via the pelvis and sacrum up to the base of the skull;
- through the foot reflexology zones, the blood supply of the organs.

Performing the exercise
Massage both feet so that it feels good, vary speed and pressure according to how you like it. Massage and stretch all the toes including their joints

gently from the root outward. Include the forefoot as well as the whole heel, the ankle and the Achilles tendon. The latter you can span with both hands along its progression, massage it with slight serpentine motions and softly stretch it.

Even if you do not know either the many reflex zone and acupressure points or the meridians, with a full foot massage you will automatically activate many of these energy points.

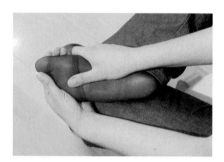 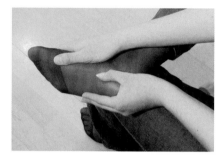

Foot massage

Relaxing the costal (rib) arch ca. 1 min.

sitting, lying down, possibly standing

Our main breathing muscle, the diaphragm, is located along the lower costal arch. A free and relaxed diaphragm helps us to breathe fully.

It holds in its tone and flexibility much knowledge about body, emotions, mind and soul. The diaphragm resonates differently to joy or delight than to crying, fear or pain. It takes on every shock but also knows how to unwind – e.g., when laughing or doing relaxed "circular breathing" (see page 45).

This self-massage promotes:
- free breathing motions in chest and belly;
- increased movement of various organs;
- permeability of the entire torso;
- purification, digestion and vitality;
- spontaneous expression, verbal and nonverbal

Performing the exercise

You run your hands along the edge of the lower costal arch from the inside out and thus relax the tissue on the surface close to the diaphragm.

1. Sitting or lying comfortably you take a few deep breaths, thereby sensing the movements of the breath going down into your pelvis. Focus and feel the ischium, your legs and feet and your connection to the earth.

2. Palpate with the fingertips of both hands how your lower costal arch runs outwards on both sides. Get to know the structure and the tone of the lower costal arch, and how it progresses. Notice how breathing moves the body continuously, expands and slightly contracts it.

3. Bring the fingers of both hands to the middle of the lower costal arch. Observe your breath flowing in and out, without changing it.

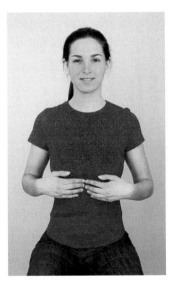
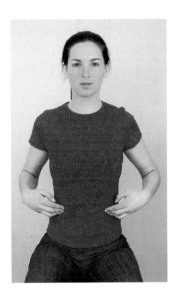

Running your hand along
the lower costal arch

The best time for running your hand along the lower costal arch is when breathing out. The next time you start breathing out, begin smoothing out the tissue along the costal arch to the left and to the right simultaneously (with the left hand following the left costal arch, the right hand following the right costal arch). After the smoothing, allow yourself several breathing cycles to feel into this sensation. In this fashion, you can run your hands along the costal arch a few times and increase or decrease the intensity of the touch.

Belly massage

sitting, lying down, possibly standing

Recent scientific findings confirm the research by Gerda Boyesen, founder of Biodynamic Body Therapy: we possess a "belly brain," which has at least as many nerve cells at its disposal as our "head brain" does. That is why we speak of "butterflies in our stomach" or "fire in our belly," or say we "can't stomach" something. When they enjoy food, children all over the world make the same movement: their hands rub their bellies in a clockwise motion. This means as much as saying: "Yum, that's good!"

This self-massage promotes:

- the relaxation of organs in the area of belly and pelvis, in particular the colon;
- the proper motion (motility) and movement (mobility) in the overall environment of the organs, the fascia and the criss-crossing connective tissue;
- the solar plexus;
- the vagus nerve with its approximately 31,000 nerve fibres rising to the brain.

Performing the exercise

1. After you have grounded and focused yourself, observe a few times how your breath flows in and out. Notice the movements of the breath in your belly, pelvis and chest.
2. Smooth along your big abdominal muscle (M. rectus abdominis) in its progression from the middle of the lower costal arch down to the pelvis.

   You begin as in the former exercise, "Relaxing the costal arch" (pages 34–35), by positioning your fingertips in the middle of the lower costal arch (fingertips signifies here the whole phalanx; this surface enables a particularly sensitive touch). You touch with a large surface of the fingers (2 to 3 phalanxes) since the big abdominal muscle that you smooth out downwards is quite big. You can repeat this smoothing out several times. It is beneficial when you follow this big muscle in its progression down to the pelvis while breathing out: you observe the phase of breathing in and then, when breathing out, you smooth from the middle of the lower costal arch in the middle of the belly plane down towards the pubic bone/pelvis, in a width of about 5 to 10 centimeters (2 to 4 inches).

3. With the whole surface of the fingers gently smooth a large area on your belly in a clockwise direction; if comfortable, you can use the whole surface of all fingers and palms. This touch is soft and follows the contours of the belly. The colon rises in the area of the belly from the bottom right up along the right side, then runs across from the right to the left, then from the top left down to the bottom left.

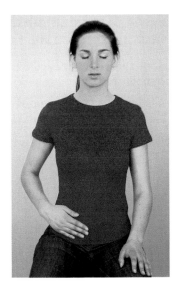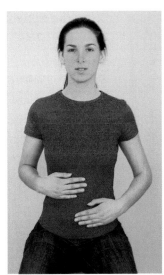

Belly massage clockwise

Place one hand on the starting point at the bottom right, above the big pelvic bone where your colon starts. Allow yourself enough time so that your hand can connect comfortably with the surface it touches at the bottom right. How does the tissue feel here?

Now begin with slow gentle and circular movements in a clockwise direction. Your hand always remains in extensive contact with the belly. Later you can increase the intensity of the touch and speed up a bit, if you wish. If this feels comfortable, continue at will with 5, 10 or 20 additional enjoyable circular movements.

At times you can also include the other hand for support. As soon as you are familiar with this sequence you can close your eyes and direct your attention to your holistic body awareness. The clockwise belly massage can occasionally be combined with smoothing out the big abdominal muscle and relaxing the costal arch.

Palpating, smoothing and massaging
the chewing muscles
ca. 3 – 10 min.

sitting, lying down, standing

The chewing muscles are particularly grateful if we relax them every now and again. They not only clench when chewing but also react to stress and express our tension by hardening. The muscles of mastication and the jaw joint mirror experiences like "biting the bullet," "biting off more than we can chew," and "facing up to something." This stress is sometimes expressed in teeth grinding. In stressful situations such as heated discussions, the high tension can virtually be seen on the side of the face in the hyper-tonus of the big chewing muscle, the masseter (M. masseter) and the temporal (M. temporalis). The masseter, which connects the lower with the upper jaw and allows us to bite, is the strongest muscle in our body – circus artists sometimes use it to carry their whole body weight! The big temporal muscle runs sideways along the head up towards the edge of the cranium (cranially).

Not only the jaw joint but also the whole craniosacral system profits from the relaxation of the chewing muscles. The big temporal muscle leads up from the lower jaw (more specifically from the coronoid process, Processus coronoideus), connects to the greater wing of sphenoid bone (Ala major), travels sideways over the frontal bone (Os frontale) and covers a large area on the parietal bone (Os parietale) and the temporal bone (Os temporale).

This self-massage promotes:
- the relaxation of the mentioned chewing muscles;
- indirectly, the relaxation of other chewing muscles, as well as ligaments and sinews affected when chewing;
- the mobility of the cranial sutures (e.g., the Sutura squamosa);
- the craniosacral rhythm of the parietal and temporal bones as well as the sphenoid bone;
- the statics of the base of the skull;
- the function of the atlanto-occipital joint.

Performing the exercise
We relax the chewing muscles through simple, conscious palpating of the tension as well as with light smoothing and massaging of these muscles, ligaments, sinews and fascia.

A) Palpating and touching the chewing muscles (temporal muscle, masseter)

1. Both muscles are very easy to palpate from the outside. Place your flat hands on the sides of your head. Position your palms sideways on lower and upper jaw, the surfaces of the fingers on the sides of your head in front of and above the ears. The thumb can reach around the auricle (outer ear) but is otherwise passive. With the surfaces of your hands and fingers you softly contact a large area of the tissue. What does this area feel like? How does it feel without additional tension of the chewing muscles? Now briefly clench your teeth about three times and palpate the tone of the masseter in the area of the jaw and of the temporal muscle in the side of the head. How do the clenched chewing muscles feel? Release all tension.

2. Relax the chewing muscles by touching the muscles on the side with both palms, afterwards slightly releasing the lower jaw. Consciously breathe out a few times the tension you experienced.

3. Invite a yawn. Once the surfaces of your palms and fingers have gentle contact with a large area on the side of the head, drop and lift the lower jaw several times softly and tenderly. Increase your breathing a bit more while doing this, continue the slow opening and closing of the lower jaw – and enjoy a copious yawn!

B) Smoothing out the chewing muscles

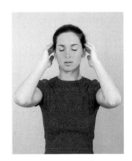

Smoothing out the temporal muscles towards the top

1. *Temporal muscle:* Softly palpate and touch a large area of the already-sensed temporal muscles with the surfaces of your fingers. Briefly clench your teeth. What does this area feel like? Now place your fingertips flat on the big temporal muscle and slowly smooth it out towards the edge of your head (cranially) with your fingertips. Repeat this smoothing out several times. While doing this let your lower jaw drop again slightly; thus you reach a multiple relaxing effect.

2. *Masseter:* With the surfaces of your fingers on both hands, simultaneously palpate the upper jaw, the masseter and the lower jaw on the sides of your head. Position your fingertips on the zygomatic arch (Arcus zygomaticus). The entire surface of your fingers makes soft, clear contact with the skin and the structure underneath (depending on the place, you feel bones, muscles or tissue underneath the layer of skin). The mas-

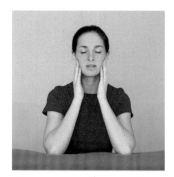

Elbows propped up: smoothing
the masseter downwards

seter is connected to the inside of the zygomatic arch and runs to the outer part of the lower jaw (Angulus mandibulae). You can easily feel it through repeated, brief clenching of your teeth. Once the surfaces of your fingers are comfortably connected with a large area of the zygomatic arch and the masseter, you slowly smooth the masseter towards the lower jaw following its general direction. As you do this, let your lower jaw slightly drop while you breathe in and out and feel how your shoulders lift and sag. Thus you make sure that you stay loose and mobile in the area of the shoulders, neck and arms.

3. Slow smoothing out/"stretching the face": Now allow yourself to continue the smoothing out even less actively. Whether you are standing or sitting, use the weight of your arms to let the surfaces of your fingers that are placed in the area of the cheeks on the side slowly slide off towards the feet (caudally). This way your palms that are connected with the masseter slowly slide down on both sides until in the end they can slip across the edge of the lower jaw. Thus you comfortably smooth out the masseter. Repeat this movement a few times. Take some time for this; observe how the surfaces of your fingers, in particular the whole area of the front phalanxes, slowly glide down and thus relax this chewing muscle in the direction it runs.

While doing this close your eyes occasionally in order to perceive the relaxation and the flow of the breath from the inside.

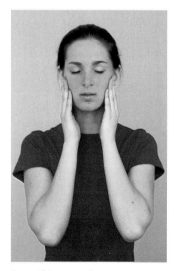
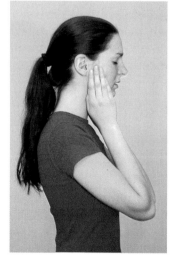
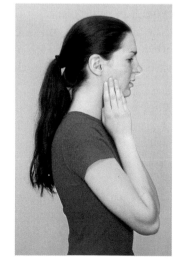

Smoothing out the masseter towards the bottom/"stretching the face"

C) Massaging the chewing muscles

Since you have already palpated and smoothed out both your temporal muscles and your masseter in their running direction, you are familiar with their exact position and tightness. Now massage the temporal muscles and the masseter along their general direction. Begin slowly and smoothly. Later you can increase and vary the intensity of the touch and speed at any time. Always stay with what feels comfortable for you. Repeat the massage a few times.

Palpating, smoothing out and massaging the outer chewing muscles can be repeated and combined as often as you like.

Hearty, copious yawning

Spontaneous yawning in between the exercises has a wonderfully releasing effect on all chewing muscles and supports relaxation in the whole body. As with relaxing, you cannot force yawning but you can invite it through letting go. Cats and dogs regulate their tension-relaxation several times a day through copious yawning, stretching and straightening, among other things – and this not only upon waking! Yawning is a natural relaxing reaction of the body. Sometimes it is accompanied by involuntary releases such as tears, coughing, sneezing, breathing again, sighing, or repeated yawning.

Scalp massage   ca. 2 – 5 min.

standing, sitting, lying down

For many people the scalp is often very tense. Those who have already received enjoyable scalp massages at the hairdresser's know how pleasurable they are and how much they assist in relaxing you. A tight, very taut scalp often points to tensions and restrictions not only in the skull but also at the base of the skull and in the area of the neck and the shoulders.

This self-massage promotes:

- a looser scalp;
- better blood circulation and purification of the scalp;
- prevention of calcification of the cranial bones and sutures;
- activation of acupuncture points of various meridians;
- more space for the fascia, ligaments and muscles connected with the scalp, in particular for the outer surface of the cranial bones and sutures; this can improve the qualities of the craniosacral rhythm.

Performing the exercise

You massage your scalp as if you were washing your hair without water (perhaps with a natural hair oil for the scalp), but more gently and slowly.

1. Feel the scalp through your hair with your fingertips. Allow yourself some time, so that the fingertips can connect well with the scalp. Then start sliding your scalp slowly and consistently slightly to the side – if possible without slipping with the fingertips at the contact point. This way you do not put any pressure on the cranium or the sutures but simply slide the scalp slightly.

2. In addition use light, small circular movements, without letting the fingertips slip. Occasionally change the positions of your fingers and thus massage the various areas of the scalp. Pay attention to the zones above the forehead, at the side of the head, at the skullcap and at the back of the head. Every now and then close your eyes while doing this, let your lower jaw drop and your breath flow.

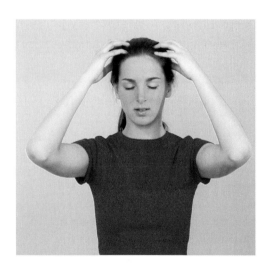
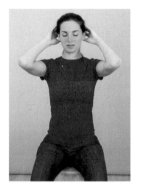

Massage of the scalp

Ear massage

ca. 2 – 5 min.

standing, sitting, lying down

Subsequent to the scalp massage, knead your auricles and earlobes with three fingers of each hand. As you do this, feel the various forms of the auricle, from the inside as well as from the outside. The light ear massage increases blood circulation and activates reflex zones.

Awareness 2 and perception exercises

Exercises for increasing body awareness

The introductory information for the following awareness and perception exercises can be found at the beginning of the exercises in the "Introduction" chapter (pages 8–10) and in "Important guidelines for treating yourself" (pages 18–27).

The self-help exercises in this part can be performed predominantly sitting or lying down. If there are some exercises that are not easy for you to carry out or do not feel comfortable, just skip them.

Breathing

The breath is our most loyal companion from the first to the last breath in our body, the temple of the soul. Our respiration is being managed by the autonomic nervous system but can also be influenced arbitrarily. Moreover, the breath mirrors our existential orientation and emotional world. It links our "inside" with the "outside."

Listen and observe consciously how the breath flows in and out.

This is one of the oldest meditations and exercises for training the consciousness. About 3,000 years ago the Buddha practised Vipassana (observing the breath as a meditation). Many meditators today also use the breath as a gateway to widening the consciousness – regardless of the respective meditation tradition or school.

In the West there are various schools of breathing – e.g., the one according to Middendorf, holotropic breathwork, rebirthing/conscious breathing. Health-enhancing practices from the East, such as Yoga or Qi Gong, use the breath as a central element in their exercises.

Sensing and observing the breath   ca. 2 – 10 min. or longer

sitting, lying down, possibly standing

Listening to the breath is a focusing exercise which often has the effect that after a while the breath becomes more even and full. The attention moves from thinking into becoming more aware of the body, so that just by itself thinking decreases to the point where thoughts only occasionally pop up. When we observe our breath we direct our awareness inside and reconnect ourselves more and more with the essence of our being.

Free breathing promotes:
- flexibility and statics in general, but particularly:
  - of the spine and the spinal dura mater,
  - of the lateral layers of connective tissue in the pelvic floor,
  - of the diaphragm,
  - of the shoulder/neck area up to the base of the skull,
  - of the muscles and ligaments of the upper aperture of the ribcage (superior thoracic aperture) up to the base of the skull;
- the flowing of the body fluids and purification;
- the functions of the organs;
- vitality.

Performing the exercise

1. Ground and center yourself. Observe your breath as it flows in and out. Let your breath flow without changing anything. Do you breathe more into the chest or into the belly?
2. Allow yourself to breathe a bit more deeply into the chest, the belly and down into the pelvis. After some fuller breaths let go of any active doing and observe your breath as it flows in and out by itself. Where in your body and how do you feel the movements of your breath?

   Every now and then close your eyes in order to perceive your breathing even better from the inside. After a while you can connect the breathing in and breathing out without any pause in between. This is also called "circular breathing" (see the following exercise).

Circular breathing
ca. 2 – 10 min. or longer

· ·

sitting, lying down

Performing the exercise

1. With circular breathing you connect breathing in and breathing out. Your breath is round and even, without any pause between breathing in and breathing out. Perhaps the inner image of a circle will help you: the first half of the circle stands for breathing in, the second half of the circle stands for breathing out.

2. Do you breathe more into the chest or into the belly? Invite yourself to breathe a bit more deeply into chest, belly and pelvis. After a few fuller breaths again let go of any active doing, move into the circular breathing and observe the in- and out-flow of the breath.

3. Occasionally you can place your hands on the area of the pelvis, belly or chest and thus give the breath more attention and space in this area.

The exercise "Relaxing the costal arch" (page 34) can be used before, during or after the circular breathing.

About the speed: slower breathing has a rather calming, grounding and centering effect. Through somewhat faster and deeper breathing, this practice can be used as an active breathing exercise for the purpose of stocking up on energy and energizing. Breathing routines can also be combined with exercises on directing energy (e.g., chakra breathing, chi/prana breathing).

Both breathing exercises are helpful for various other self-treatments:

- as preparation;
- in between other exercises;
- combined with other exercises;
- as time for gathering yourself in between the exercises, in order to perceive the differences (before-after).

No matter whether you listen to the breath
or to the craniosacral rhythm: both can serve as meditation!

Resources: to connect yourself
consciously with power sources   any duration

standing, sitting, lying down

Resources are inner and outer sources of power on which we can rely for renewed strength, confidence and self-confidence in good times as well as in troubled times or situations. Every person experiences and defines their sources of power individually. Inner resources consist of, for example:

- a basic trust in life;
- strong faith;
- spontaneity, openness to the new;
- equanimity.

Outer resources could include:

- nature;
- our life partner or very good friends;
- pets;
- hobbies.

Those who connect with their inner and outer resources can experience how the mood and the sense of the body change. This is an empowering exercise as our resources influence directly, partly automatically, our thoughts and feelings and ultimately how we sense and experience our body.

Being in contact with our resources means not to see the glass as half empty but to see it as half full. You have survived even difficult times – and in most cases those times could have been worse. What was it then that made you strong enough to persevere successfully?

A body part or an area of the body that feels very good and comfortable to you can also be a resource.

Performing the exercise

1. Ground and center yourself, observing your breath as it flows in and out. Now remember:
   - a beautiful encounter;
   - an impressive nature experience; or
   - the most recent joyful message you received.

2. Perceive what changes in you physically as you think about or connect with this experience, this power source. Feel, for example, how your breathing becomes more relaxed and full, or how the posture, the muscle tension, the sensation of warmth and the expression of the face change.

3. Stay with your memory, your power source, and the feeling connected with it. With eyes open or closed, sense where your body feels comfortable, relaxed, spacious, warm, pleasurable. Allow yourself time so that this new body feeling can deepen and expand. You support this by placing one or both hands on the particular part of the body where you feel the change. Keep your attention in that area of the body. If applicable, move with the same attention to other regions of the body that have also relaxed.

Occasionally connect with your resources, in everyday life as well as before and during the self-treatments. If, for example, you have deeply and comfortably felt your belly in the area of the navel a few times, you can remember this and focus in difficult situations on your belly.

Sensing feet, legs, pelvis, sacrum: grounding, centering, connecting

ca. 2 – 5 min.

sitting, lying down, standing

Performing the exercise

Move your attention to the lower half of your body. Ground and center yourself and feel the connection of your feet and legs with the pelvis and the sacrum. Become aware of the unit that the lower part of your body forms. During the exercise let your connected breath flow (without pause between in- and out-breath) and slightly drop the lower jaw.

1. Feel your feet and where they touch the floor or other surface. Do your feet feel light or heavy, warm or cool, spacious or restricted? Give the weight of your feet to the earth.

2. Feel your legs and their connection through your feet to the earth. Do your legs feel light or heavy, warm or cool, spacious or restricted? Give the weight of your legs to the earth.

3. Feel the whole of your pelvis:

- where it touches the surface;
- where and how much weight of the pelvis is given to the base upon which it is resting;
- the right and left sides of the pelvis;
- the pubic bone with the symphysis in the middle;
- your sacrum that links the spine with the pelvis;
- the whole area of the pelvis, three-dimensionally, spatially.

Now feel your pelvis again connected with your legs, feet and the whole surface. Consciously give your weight down, trust the earth with it.

You remain in the flow of the breath, the mouth slightly open.
- How do you perceive your body structure?
- How do you sense your skin, your muscles, your bones, your joints?

With increasing experience you will be able to distinguish between these different body layers and then return to the holistic body awareness (see page 59).

4. Move your attention again to your sacrum, which you have already palpated in the area of the pelvis. Become aware of the whole bony structure of this "sacred bone" (= Os sacrum). Feel the connecting surface of the sacrum:
   - upwards towards the spine, to the lowest lumbar vertebra (lumbosacral joint, L5-S1);
   - sideways to the hip bones (sacroiliac joint).

5. While you perceive your sacrum holistically, simultaneously feel your whole inner pelvic area, the ischium and the hips, the legs and the feet. Remain grounded, centered and in holistic body awareness as long as you like. At the end take a few deep breaths, perhaps stretch or straighten yourself a bit or yawn.

Sensing sacrum, spine and their connection to the occipital bone   ca. 2 min.

sitting, lying down, possibly standing

The connection between sacrum, spine and occipital bone is of central importance for the craniosacral system. The spinal dura mater (Dura mater spinalis), which covers and protects the medulla, is fastened at the great foramen magnum, in the area of the 2nd/3rd cervical (C2/3) and at the sacrum (at S2). The craniosacral rhythm is being transmitted via the occipital bone, the connective tissue and the spinal dura mater downwards to the sacrum and the pelvis.

The part of the atlas (the first cervical vertebra) that points towards the head, along with the occipital condyles, constitutes the atlanto-occipital joint and forms the bony transition to the skull and the base of the skull.

The statics of the spinal dura mater also influence the statics of the intracranial membranes and thus the whole cranium.

Both the sacrum and the occipital bone have many extra parasympathetic nerve fibres. As you listen to, observe and gently touch these zones, your parasympathetic nervous system is strengthened.

Performing the exercise

Move your attention to pelvis and sacrum. Ground and center yourself the way you did in the previous exercise.

1. Palpate your pelvis, in particular the sacrum. Does it feel light or heavy, warm or cool, spacious or restricted? Let go of its weight downwards. Continue to let your breath flow freely and let the lower jaw drop slightly.

2. While you palpate your sacrum, begin to slowly move your attention along the lumbar spine, vertebra by vertebra. Allow yourself enough time to palpate each vertebra, one at a time. After the lumbar vertebrae, greet and palpate each individual thoracic vertebra, then each cervical vertebra. Be sure to allow extra time for the first cervical vertebra in order to really feel into this region.

3. Now palpate your occipital bone, the area of the back of your head, and the lower edge of the cranium. Any tensions that you feel in this region you now breathe out through a slightly-opened mouth. How do sacrum, spine and occipital bone feel now? What feels light or heavy, warm or cool, spacious or restricted?

4. Now feel the whole pelvic area including legs and feet (grounded), the sacrum, the spine, the occipital bone, the entire head. Again allow yourself extra time to palpate the first cervical, the transition to the cranium, in order to really sense this region.

   Perceive yourself now as a whole, three-dimensional and spatial. Release your weight downwards. Remain for a few minutes without tension in this holistic body awareness.

Sensing ribcage, shoulder blades, shoulders, arms, cervical spine, head

ca. 2 – 5 min.

grounding, centering, connecting
sitting, lying down, possibly standing

Performing the exercise

Now we include the upper extremities:

1. Become aware of your pelvis, the sacrum and the spine, as in the preceding exercise. Ground and center yourself.
2. Stay connected with pelvis and sacrum and move your inner attention slowly up the spine.
3. When you reach the thoracic spine take your time to palpate as many as possible of the ribs attached to the sides of the vertebrae, including the costal arch. Become aware of the whole chest area, how it widens when breathing in and decreases in size when breathing out.
4. Perceive the front of the bony thorax, including both collarbones (clavicles). Become aware of the back side of the bony thorax, including both shoulder blades (scapulas). Also palpate both arms and hands, down to the fingertips (the whole surface of the top phalanx).
5. Release all tension. Palpate your whole ribcage and shoulder/neck area including cervical spine and occipital bone or the back of the head:
    *   How does it feel in the individual areas mentioned?
    *   Where does it feel light, where heavy?
    *   Where does it feel warm or cool?
    *   Where does it feel spacious or restricted?
    *   Where does it feel particularly comfortable?

Feel the whole region as one unit. Consciously release your weight downward. Continue to let your breath flow freely and let your lower jaw drop slightly.

With your inner attention connect the whole shoulder/neck area with the spine, the sacrum, the pelvis and the feet. Ground and center yourself. Now perceive yourself from head to toe as a whole, three-dimensionally. Remain for another few minutes in this holistic body awareness. Then finish this exercise by lightly stretching, straightening and yawning.

Sensing individual body parts

30 sec. – 5 min.
variable according to body part

sitting, lying down, possibly standing

In the preceding exercises you have already listened to the movement of the breath and have grounded and centered yourself as well as perceived pelvic, spine and shoulder/neck areas up to the head. Coming away from your holistic body awareness, direct your attention now to individual body parts of your choice.

Performing the exercise

1. You ground and center yourself and let your breath flow freely.
2. Palpate, for example, your arms and hands, your bones and feet, your pelvis including sacrum, further body structures such as breastbone (sternum), jaw joint, diaphragm.

Perceiving organs and relaxing them through touch

ca. 1 – 5 min. per organ

sitting, lying down

With this exercise you can broaden your awareness and also direct your attention to individual organs. Choose to sense the liver, the gallbladder, the spleen, the uterus or prostate, the lobes of the lung or your heart. By touching the body part gently, making conscious contact and inviting space and expanse, you deepen the relaxation of that organ as you deepen your ability to perceive and sense.

Craniosacral practitioners treat these organs with one or several visceral treatments.

Perceiving, relaxing and connecting body segments and segment transitions

ca. 1 – 5 min.
or more

sitting, lying down, possibly standing

The seven body segments according to Wilhelm Reich (eyes, mouth, neck, chest, diaphragm, belly, pelvis) are characterized by different physical functions as well as different psycho-emotional topics. In contrast to armored (tense) segments, free body segments linked with each other can allow life energy to flow better throughout the body. Spontaneous expression, creativity and joy are being supported or encumbered, depending on the tension in and between the individual segments.

Gerda Boyesen named the line arising from belly and chest via throat to mouth and eyes the "Id channel" or "It channel" (the channel of expressing the "it," our primary personality), while John E. Upledger speaks about it as the "avenue of expression."

These awareness and sensing exercises support and promote:

- organs and adenoids which are being assisted in their function, directly or indirectly;
- perceiving the body as a whole;
- relaxing the musculoskeletal system.

The "belly brain" notifies the "head brain" on the neurological and the endocrine level of the increased relaxation, which has positive effects on various body functions.

With regular exercise and a bit of patience, different layers of the body can be differentiated and discerned – e.g., the layers of the skin, of the connective tissue and muscles or of the bones. After perceiving them individually you reconnect with your holistic body awareness.

Performing the exercise (goes for all positions)

Tender touch and gentle approach with our hands to individual body segments brings more space and expanse to these and enhances bodily awareness.

Place your hand or both hands on the chosen segment. You can choose and relax an individual segment or several segments. The instructions show how you can relax them step-by-step from bottom to top; it is also possible to do it the other way around. Afterwards you will see possibilities for connecting the segments with each other.

1. Gently touch the chosen body segment with relaxed hands. The surfaces of hands and fingers should touch as much of the area as possible – just as if your hand is allowing itself to be molded by the underlying perceivable structure – without any tension in hands, fingers or wrists. Occasionally close your eyes in order to direct your attention inside.
2. Have your "palpation awareness" work for you: The soft touch allowing spaciousness and the warmth of your hands and fingers relax the structure as much on its surface as deep within.
   - What does this area feel like?

- Does anything change when you breathe into this segment a few times from within?
- What do you feel under your hands?
- What does this touch feel like inside?

The tension is not being broken by invasive manual techniques but is being softened, dissolved by "consciousness through touch." You accept the tension as a natural limit and wait with conscious and coherent touch until the tissue under your hands has relaxed by itself.

Relaxing the segments and their transitions is similar to relaxing the connective tissue (Part 3, pages 89), which constitutes a significant continuation of the segment treatments described here. There you will find further information about the quality of touch and more specifically about what these relaxations promote.

The pelvic segment

ca. 1 – 5 min. or longer

sitting, lying down

Place the whole surface of your hands on the pelvis. If you touch with one hand, place it with its full surface across. Two hands are preferably positioned in the form of a V: the little fingers are placed in the area of the groin, and the fingertips are positioned above the pubic bone in order to contact as much surface of the pelvic segment as possible.

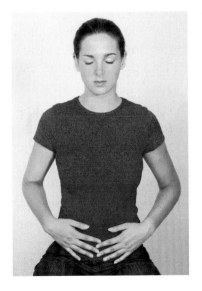

Touching the pelvic segment

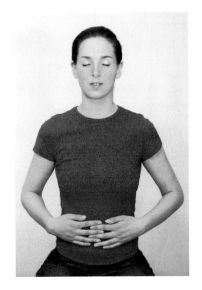

Touching the belly segment

The belly segment

ca. 1 – 5 min. or longer

sitting, lying down

Place the whole surface of your hands on the belly. Position the thumbs directly underneath the costal arch. The fingers can be slightly spread and placed next to each other in such a way that you have comprehensive contact with the surface. Once you have palpated and relaxed the tissue of the belly segment in this place for a while, you can change the hand positions according to your own discretion:

- slightly deeper, towards the pelvic segment;
- slightly higher, the surfaces of the thumbs on the costal arch;
- sideways (the two hands do not touch each other any longer then), in order to become aware of the whole belly area between your hands and to let it expand and become more spacious.

The diaphragm segment

ca. 1 – 5 min. or longer

sitting, lying down

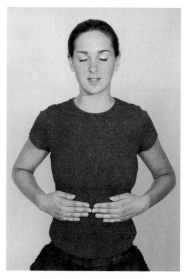

Touching the segment of the diaphragm/lower costal arch

The segment of the diaphragm, the area of the lower costal arch including the solar plexus, carries a special importance (also see "Relaxing the costal arch," pages 34). This is where the statics of the upper and lower torso meet. Often our body attempts to clear an imbalance in the area of the pelvis or shoulder/neck via the diaphragm segment.

Place the whole surface of your hands horizontally on your lower costal arch. The fingers can be slightly spread and placed within each other or with only the middle fingers touching, as the photo shows. This way you also touch the upper part of the belly. Feel the rhythm of your breath underneath your hands and invite spaciousness. As you do this, relax the shoulder/neck area. Breathe out tensions through the slightly-opened mouth.

The chest segment   ca. 1 – 5 min. or longer

sitting, lying down

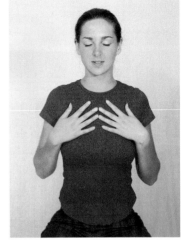

1. Place the entire palm of both hands on the upper chest area. If you contact with one hand only, this hand can be positioned horizontally with the full surface of the palm touching, across the breastbone (sternum). Through the clothes, using the surfaces of your hands and fingers, connect gently with the layer of skin and the upper tissue of the chest.

2. By increasing the intensity of your touch, establish contact with the level of the bones, with the various ribs and the breastbone. Are you well connected there? Have you experienced this area from the inside, too?

Touching the chest segment

3. With a bit of practice and slightly more intense touch you can also become aware of the area behind the costal arch. Repeated deep breathing into the chest segment provides additional relaxation there.

The throat and neck segment   ca. 1 – 5 min. or longer

sitting, lying down

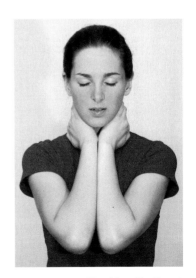

Place your hands slowly, gently and with as much surface of the palm as possible on your throat and neck area. The wrists are in contact with each other and thus lend stability in order to be able to touch calmly and evenly. With your hands and fingers touch as much surface of your throat and neck as possible. Once your hands are linked without pressure, give the whole contacted structure more space. Especially here in the throat and neck segment – slender and narrow compared to other body segments – we take great care with our touch in order not to have a constricting effect.

Closing your eyes, palpate your neck between the hands and invite spaciousness. Release your shoulder/neck area. Breathe out tensions through your slightly-opened mouth.

Touching the throat and neck segment

The mouth segment

ca. 1 – 5 min. or longer

sitting, lying down

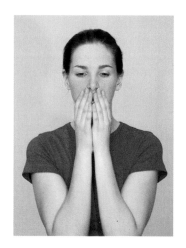

Place your ring fingers, middle fingers and index fingers so that they touch the whole area around your mouth extensively. When you use two hands, the little fingers are not involved, and the tips of the ring fingers touch above the mouth. Your fingertips contact as much of the surface of your lips and the skin around your mouth as possible, gently and without pressure. Now allow the whole contacted structure more space. Your lower jaw is allowed to drop slightly; the relaxed lips facilitate breathing out via a slightly-opened mouth.

Touching the mouth segment

The eyes segment

ca. 1 – 5 min. or longer

sitting, lying down

In everyday life the eyes fulfill an important control function, among others. Seeing is mostly focused. The eyes observe with concentration; they are often like a hunter on the prowl for something. This is why bioenergetics and vision exercises always work with the eye segment. Through closing our eyes, touching ourselves gently around the eyes and listening within, a rigid, armored eye segment often relaxes by itself. Closing your eyes, directing your gaze within and then sensing is one of the simplest and oldest meditations.

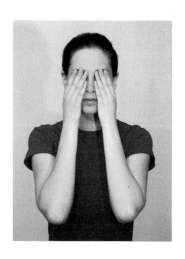

Performing the exercise

Place the surfaces of your fingers above the closed eyes, covering a large area. The fingertips of the index, middle and ring fingers are positioned on the eyebrows or slightly higher. Instead of the fingers you can also place your palms across the area of your eyes – choose whichever feels more comfortable for you. Underneath the eyes you gently touch the cheekbones (zygomatic bone/Os zygomaticum). The eyeballs are not being touched; they can recede slightly into the eye sockets. Release all tension in the whole area of the eyes.

Touching the eye segment

Connecting and relaxing body segments
and segment transitions
ca. 1 – 5 min. or longer

sitting, lying down

After you have perceived and relaxed the individual body segments in detail, contact different segments or segment transitions with both hands respectively at the same time. Segment transitions – areas that link two segments with each other – deserve particular attention. It depends on their statics or their permeability whether this zone is separating or connecting.

**There are several ways to connect and relax
two segments at the same time:**

- From the bottom to the top, in ascending order, start with pelvis, then belly (when changing, place the lower hand on the next free segment – i.e., the hands keep moving up in turns).
- One hand always remains connected with a segment – e.g., with the pelvis or diaphragm/costal arch – while the second hand touches the other segments or segment transitions step-by-step and moves upwards.
- Remember the segment that you have perceived to be the most comfortable one. Place one hand on it, the second directly underneath or above. Consciously connect with this source of power. From this spot the sense of well-being can expand upwards and downwards.

We recommend using the ascending order, but you do not need to follow any fixed sequence. You can also intuitively touch a body segment or a segment transition of your choice with one hand, then the next one with the other hand.

You tune into: quality of the touch, clear and gentle connection with the segment, listening, giving space, inviting expanse. Sense the movements of the breath and release your lower jaw, the weight and all tensions.

When you simultaneously relax two segments that are not directly adjoining, move your attention occasionally not only to the contacted segments but also to the area between those segments:

- Does anything change there? If so, what and how?
- Can you feel a connection between the two touched segments?

Simultaneous boost of the activity of the glands and the chakra balance

ca. 1 – 5 min. or longer

sitting, lying down

In the area around all segments, contacting and relaxing them addresses essential parts of the body, such as gonads, adrenal glands, solar plexus and pancreas, stomach, thymus gland, thyroid, pituitary and pineal glands.

These areas are directly or closely connected to the chakras (Sanskrit for "wheel"). These transformational centers of vibrating energy allow an exchange of energy between body, environment and cosmos.

Touching and relaxing the segments simultaneously harmonizes the chakras, the seven etheric energy centers of our body:

- the base chakra in the pelvis (1);
- the hara in the belly/navel area (2);
- the solar plexus under the costal arch/diaphragm (3);
- the heart chakra in the area of the chest (4);
- the throat chakra in the area of the throat/neck (5);
- the third eye in the area of the eyes, between the eyebrows (6);
- the crown chakra in the area of the vertex (top of head) (7).

As you treat the segments, you harmonize the chakras in the area of the torso. For example:

1. grounded and centered, you first touch the transition between pelvis-belly (hara);
2. then the costal arch/diaphragm (solar plexus);
3. then the breastbone and the chest (heart chakra);
4. then the eyes and the forehead (third eye),
5. possibly combined with touching the sagittal suture (crown chakra).

Treatment of the segments can be enhanced by placing both hands on one chakra or with various hand positions on different chakras at the same time.

Holistic body awareness
any duration

Perceiving the body in its wholeness
sitting, lying down, possibly standing

Whether you perform the exercises from Part 1, 2 or 3, go with your resources and direct your attention first towards those body parts that feel
pleasurable. Deep breathing often facilitates local relaxation which expands
to other body segments and levels.

Feel the areas that are loosening up, not in isolation but in the wholeness of your body, allowing the places you use as resources to expand even
further. Fully enjoy this holistic body awareness.

In this way important neurological structures – like the amygdaloid body
(Corpus amygdaloideum) that records and remembers conditions of excitement and fear – receive new information of deep relaxation and letting
go. Feeling whole and in connection with the inner source allows us to rest
in our center. Our peripheral alarm sensors are mostly switched off. There
is no need for defense.

With steady practice you will find it increasingly easy to switch between
detailed perception of individual (comfortable) body parts and the holistic
body awareness in which you feel your body as a whole.

3 Harmonizing the craniosacral system

Promoting self-regulation and deep relaxation

Most of the self-help exercises in this part can be performed sitting or lying down. Palpating and treating yourself as well as receiving treatments by professional craniosacral practitioners can support your craniosacral system. In most cases, the craniosacral rhythm and its qualities are less restricted and more balanced after the self-treatment. This enhances the self-regulation and boosts the self-healing powers of the body.

In order to achieve an optimal relaxation effect with the following craniosacral exercises, please read the chapters "Introduction" (page 8) and "Important guidelines for treating yourself" (page 18) in this book. As mentioned earlier, I recommend exercises from Parts 1 and 2 as preparation.

Self-palpation

Trust your hands and your senses. You can rediscover your hands and their receiving presence as a sensitive instrument that is tuned and trained further each time you feel into and palpate your body. With the following exercise we move into resonance with our slow body rhythms, train an observing, non-judgmental perception and thereby are able to experience a natural expansion of awareness.

If you do not feel the craniosacral rhythm when you first start palpating, allow yourself some time. Often the craniosacral rhythm becomes noticeable when you listen with your hands in an absolutely relaxed space, with no goal whatsoever. You do not even need to concentrate. At the beginning you may feel slow and subtle movements for a few seconds; otherwise just enjoy the relaxation. The more often or longer you palpate yourself, the more you will feel and the more detailed your perceptions will become.

Perceiving and differentiating body rhythms: the rhythm of the breath, pulsation of the heart, craniosacral rhythm

ca. 5 – 15 min. or longer

sitting, lying down
sitting: your hands touch the thighs extensively
lying down: your hands touch the sides of the pelvis extensively

Performing the exercise

1. Place your hands gently on your thighs (sitting) or on the sides of your pelvis (lying). You do not use any pressure here but create contact with what you perceive underneath your hands. Feel your hands' weight, the muscles of your forearms, the arms, and the shoulders. Pass the weight of your body including pelvis, legs and feet into the ground, so that you need to hold as little tension as possible. Ground and center yourself. You can close your eyes and listen inwardly. There is nothing to do for the next few minutes. Allow your breathing to flow freely. Let your lower jaw slowly drop and breathe out through your slightly-open mouth.

2. Move your whole attention into your hands; feel the area of contact with your thighs or pelvis. Release any pressure in your touch; there is no need for pressure in a connected state. Thus the touch becomes even gentler. With your sensing awareness let your hands become one with the palpated area, as if the hands' receptors slide by themselves into the depth of the thigh or the sides of the pelvis and latch on until your hands and the palpated body part form a unit.

   Or:

   You may choose the reverse sequence: you touch even more gently and invite the touched structures underneath your hands to extend towards your hands, to expand.

3. *Rhythm of the breath:* Direct your attention to the breath that flows by itself in and out of your body, forming the breathing rhythm. Do not attempt to change the breath but stay attentive, observing how "it breathes." For a while watch the rhythm of your breath and whatever else might arise or develop.
   - Where in your body do you feel the rhythm of your breath?
   - Do your shoulders lift slightly when breathing in and drop again when breathing out? Perhaps the breath moves the structure of your torso including the pelvic area?
   - Do you sense the flowing in and out of the breath as rhythm in several places of the body simultaneously – or where your hands touch the body?

4. *Detailed awareness training:* You might hardly perceive the rhythm of your breath with your hands; instead you might perceive warmth, expansion, heaviness or lightness. Or you might feel the "therapeutic pulse" (see page 74) – for example, twitching of the muscles, a throbbing and pulsing. Just observe this and continue to keep your full attention where your hands touch, without changing anything.

5. *Heartbeat:* Direct your attention to your heartbeat:
   - Where do you feel it?
   - In the left side of your chest or more towards the middle?
   - In the forearms or wrists?
   - In the area of your throat or neck?
   - Do you also feel your heartbeat where your hands touch?

   You may feel it only occasionally; just enjoy lingering passively and indulge in a few minutes of stillness. Relaxed as you are, observe how your hands touch gently and without pressure. Allow yourself to lighten your touch even more.

6. *Breath and heartbeat:* It may be possible for you to feel the movement of the breath and the heartbeat at the same time. You can train yourself in consciously directing your attention slowly and alternately to the movements of your breath and then to your heartbeat – or sensing both at the same time.

7. *Craniosacral rhythm:* Move your attention to a slow, subtle movement in the body. On thighs and sides of the pelvis you might feel a minimal expansion, as the tissue turns slowly and steadily outwards, in a light outward rotating motion. This outward motion is generally followed by an inward rotating motion. It is possible that this slow rhythm stops briefly and then the tissue continues to move in the same direction, or

that after a short stop the rhythm moves the tissue in the reverse direction.

At the sides of the pelvis the slow outward rotation will feel like a lateral expansion, as if the volume inside the pelvic area is increasing. The inside rotation, on the other hand, moves the thighs or rather the iliac crests slightly to the middle, which feels as though the volume inside the pelvic area is decreasing. This is probably the craniosacral rhythm with its subtle movements of about 6 to 12 cycles per minute, slow like tidal ebb and flow. While you are listening into your body there is nothing to achieve. Allow yourself time to train the awareness of your hands.

8. *Rhythm of breath, heart and craniosacral rhythm:* Now let yourself be met by individual body rhythms that you have experienced and observe without judgment whether it is the rhythm of your breath, your heartbeat or the craniosacral rhythm that you sense. The more often you perform this exercise, the more you will feel and the easier it will be for you to direct your attention consciously and alternately to the rhythm of the breath (about 16 times per minute), the heart (about 70 to 90 times per minute) and the craniosacral system (about 6 to 12 times per minute), and listen to them. With a bit of practice it is possible to sense the different movements and body rhythms alternately or simultaneously.

9. You finish this exercise by unhurriedly bringing the sensing awareness of your hands back from inside the tissue until you again perceive the layer of the skin or your clothes underneath your hand. Take a few deep breaths, open your eyes and become aware of your outer surroundings. Slowly release the physical contact of your hands.

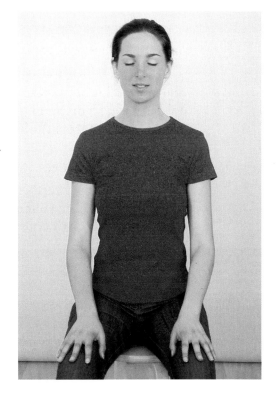

Listening to body rhythms on your thighs

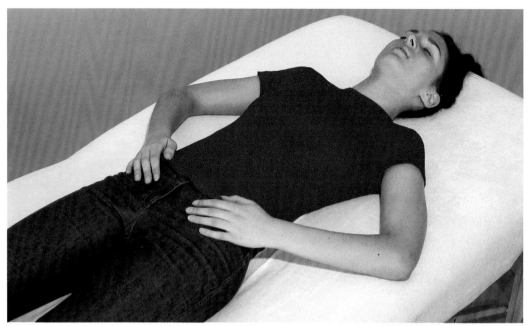

Listening to body rhythms on the sides of your pelvis

10. Now allow yourself enough time to gently and pleasurably stretch, straighten and yawn. Open your eyes and return to the world of everyday life:

- How does your whole body feel now ?
- Are there differences after doing the exercise?

Slowly take a few steps:

- What has changed inside yourself?
- How is the pattern of your gait now?
- With your senses, do you perceive changes in the "outside"? If so, what are they?

Listening to the craniosacral rhythm or slower rhythms on thighs, sides of the pelvis and head   ca. 5 – 15 min. or longer

sitting, lying down

The position on the thighs or sides of the pelvis as well as the quality of touch and performance of this self-palpation are the same as described in "Perceiving and differentiating body rhythms" (page 61). This exercise is the best introduction for listening to the craniosacral rhythm and possibly even slower rhythms.

Relaxed listening and an increasingly differentiated awareness of your body enable you to observe the craniosacral rhythm with its qualities and the alternating tidal motions more and more easily and precisely.

Having perceived and differentiated various body rhythms before, the following explanations will help you to expand and deepen your field of awareness.

Training for differentiated perception

You may not feel the craniosacral rhythm with your hands right away but instead the rhythm of your breath or your heartbeat. Just notice this, without changing anything.

- Where in your body do you feel the rhythm of your breath?
- Where most strongly, where most lightly – possibly even where your hands touch?
- Is its speed changing?
- Do you feel parallel to your breathing rhythm a slower movement in your hands or in the body?
- What else do you feel?
- What is the texture of the tissue underneath your hands?
- Do you feel more warmth or coolness?
- Does it tingle after a while?
- Does it get soft?
- Do you feel body connections, the flowing of energy? Do you perceive yourself as a whole?

More and more, not only are you connected with the layers of the skin, connective tissue and bones, but also you extend your field of awareness to the levels of the meninges of the brain and the spine, and to the fluid level of the cerebrospinal liquor, the fluid of the brain and spinal cord. Thus you automatically support and promote contact with the slow tidal movements of the craniosacral rhythm.

As you become more experienced in palpating sensitively you may find that you follow the suggested order within the exercises more loosely: you start observing a wide range of perceptions that you can deepen according to your own preferences.

Listening to the craniosacral rhythm at the head

Having a base – a table, for example – for the elbows can support comfortable self-palpation at the head, as you can then gently touch your head with your hands while your forearms are propped up. Make sure that the base is not too high or too low; books or a blanket folded accordingly can serve well to ensure this.

Palpating at the head without the mentioned base is also possible, when you are, for example, already grounded and centered through the exercises in Part 1 and 2, and have let go of all unnecessary tensions in the shoulder/neck area. Your breath is also allowed to flow freely. This assists in palpating the pelvis and the shoulder/neck area in a relaxed way, without tension.

The following photos demonstrate the touching of the frontal bone (Os frontale). You can also palpate the craniosacral rhythm and slower tidal movements on different cranial bones. This will be explained on pages 99–101 & 105–117. The illustrations and photos there can support you, as you perform the exercises, in being able to touch and listen accurately.

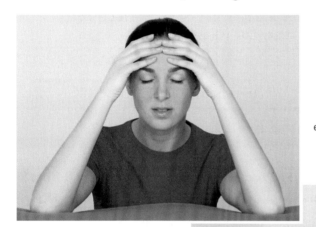

Palpating craniosacral rhythm
on frontal bone

elbows propped up

sitting

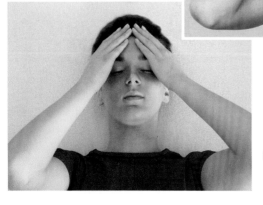

lying down

The craniosacral rhythm

Up to now I have set aside any comprehensive explanation of the craniosacral rhythm in the body. The reason for this was to enable you to experience the preceding palpation exercises with as little prejudice as possible and to trust your own perceptions. Now that you have some knowledge of palpations, we want to observe the craniosacral rhythm and the slower tidal rhythms more closely.

There are various explanation models of how the craniosacral rhythm develops. Some have a biomechanical functional background, others an energetic biodynamic one. Many skeptics continue to doubt the craniosacral rhythm or the movements of the cranial bones, but within the past 40 years the rhythm has been measured repeatedly, and with different methods. Even the change in the blood sugar during a stillpoint (when the craniosacral rhythm stops for about 30 seconds to about 4 minutes) could be verified.

Practiced lay people can palpate the craniosacral rhythm. When several craniosacral practitioners simultaneously palpate a person's body, there often is amazingly congruent feedback about the person's physical condition. You will find more about craniosacral treatment from a professional practitioner on page 130, as well as in my reference book *Craniosacral Rhythm: A practical guide to a gentle form of bodywork therapy* (Elsevier, 2008) and further technical literature as listed in the Appendix.

New cerebrospinal fluid, the Liquor cerebrospinalis, is constantly produced in the choroid plexus of the four connected cerebral ventricles. This fluid is being directed into the outer liquor cisterns at the fourth ventricle, in the area of the occipital bone (Os occipitale). One theory states that the accumulation of the cerebrospinal fluid induces the cerebrospinal fluid pressure to rise. This stretches the cerebral meninges and thus the directly connected cranial bones, in particular on their cranial sutures. In the membrane system of the spinal meninges the fluid is spread within the spinal dura mater along the spinal cord, down to the sacrum.

The craniosacral rhythm can be felt at the cranium, the spine and the sacrum, as well as in the bones and muscles and above all in the connective tissue all over the body.

Movements and qualities of the craniosacral rhythm

Progressive anatomists and traditional practitioners share with craniosacral practitioners and osteopaths the opinion that the cranial sutures do not necessarily solidly adhere when growing older but allow subtle movements like, for example, the craniosacral rhythm. These movements, in the range of micromillimeters, can be felt with practice and patience by skilled hands.

Outer and inner rotation / Movements of flexion and extension

For general self-treatment it is not necessarily required to understand this terminology, but it can be of benefit. Engaging with this highly interesting field opens up new horizons and often promotes a deepened bodily and sensory awareness. You get to know your body and its inherent intelligence anew. Informed, knowing palpation of the movements develops your detailed perception and differentiation.

When the cerebrospinal fluid pressure in the craniosacral system increases, this can be perceived as an expansion, as a becoming fuller and larger, and *in paired/outer body parts* (like on the thighs) as *outer rotation*. When the volume of the fluid in the craniosacral system decreases, this slow movement can be perceived on paired body parts as *inner rotation*.

In contrast to this, the filling and expanding of the craniosacral system – including the outer rotation that can be felt on paired body parts – is defined as *flexion at the bones of the midline* (sacrum, occiput, sphenoid bone, ethmoid bone, vomer); the decreasing is defined as *extension*. Explained biomechanically, this definition results from viewing the movements of *the base of the skull from below*.

The flexion-extension movement is carried via the occipital bone and the spinal dura mater into the whole torso where subsequently the craniosacral rhythm can be perceived as outer and inner rotation.

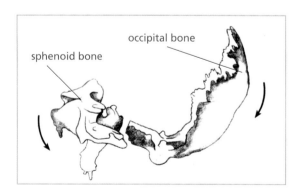

Sphenoid and occipital bones and their direction
of movement in flexion

**The four most important quality characteristics
of the craniosacral rhythm:**

- Cycles per minute: The craniosacral rhythm moves in a cycle of about 6 to 12 times per minute, slower than the rhythm of the heart and the breath. You can perceive even slower rhythms: see pages 71–72.
- Amplitude/scope: The craniosacral rhythm can display an expansive, wide area of the outer-inner rotation (OIR) flexion and extension movement or a rather narrow, restricted area. There are people with distinctively more flexion/OR or more extension/IR movement.
- Intensity: The craniosacral rhythm can be only very faintly or very intensely discernible. The intensity of the craniosacral rhythm expresses much about the present vitality and self-regulation ability of the organism.
- Symmetry left-right/harmony: You can perceive the craniosacral rhythm evenly on both sides of the body, or with more movement on the side that is less restricted.

These qualities can be perceived differently on various body parts, indicating free or restricted body structures. This is how craniosacral practitioners receive information on correlations throughout the body.

When your sensitive hands become aware of the craniosacral rhythm, listen mindfully to its slow movements. Observe throughout several cycles how these four quality characteristics express themselves and whether they change through palpating.

Do they change before, during or after the palpations, the self-treatments and the relaxation of the craniosacral system? If so, how?

Tips for differentiated palpation of the craniosacral rhythm

The craniosacral rhythm can be seen as a dynamic expression of life force. At any time the direction of the movement can change and the tidal motion can gather speed or slow down. Both can happen spontaneously, after a brief stop or a stillpoint. It can feel like two outer rotation movements happening successively before another inner rotation movement begins.

Sometimes the craniosacral rhythm feels staccato instead of flowing or can only be sensed on the left or on the right. Next to outer-inner rotation fluctuations running laterally you can simultaneously find fluctuations running longitudinally: these can be perceived as slow movements towards the head and the feet (as flexion or extension).

Inner attitude and intention when palpating:

It can happen that you expect or want to achieve too much. This creates a subtle tension on the mental, physical and energetic level, which impedes the palpation of the craniosacral rhythm. You can often sense the craniosacral rhythm when your active part has surrendered and only the observer with its open, receiving attitude remains.

Should you hardly feel anything, just enjoy remaining passive for a while and allow yourself a few minutes of gathering yourself. You may perceive differences, but do not judge the craniosacral rhythm. Follow it with a basically passive, attentive and open attitude. Engage with the subtle tidal movements that can change at any time. They always express themselves directly, in the present moment.

While palpating make a mental note of certain tendencies – for example, the qualities of the craniosacral rhythm, or rather, whether the movements become larger, clearer, more harmonious. The craniosacral movements are slow. With inner calmness and centeredness – as in meditation – and some practice, even beginners can distinctly perceive the craniosacral rhythm. You best sense the slow movements of the craniosacral rhythm when you slow down yourself and listen patiently. Many beginners feel the rhythm for the first time or particularly clearly when they have surrendered the "wish to achieve something" (see above).

Your mental attitude affects it, too. Give your "inner skeptic" or "fearmonger" a break during the self-treatments. If you drive a vehicle, operate a computer or attune to the idiosyncrasies of pets, you also need time and patience. Even when the new concepts appear strange to start with, trust that the craniosacral rhythm will appear and listen to the sensations in your hands.

You best perceive the craniosacral rhythm in a space of relaxed, observing awareness. You cannot "catch it." Let the craniosacral rhythm come to you! What do you feel underneath your gently touching, relaxed hands?

The more you practice these self-treatments and self-palpations the more you sharpen your awareness of subtle rhythms. With clear intention and gentle touch you generally support the craniosacral rhythm, regardless of whether you are presently able to palpate it or not.

Differentiating among various slower rhythms

About 100 years ago, the founder of Cranial Osteopathy, William G. Sutherland, discovered the "cranial breath," the craniosacral rhythm with about 6 to 12 cycles per minute, and named it the "primary respiratory mechanism" (PRM). He used a biomechanical explanatory model. During the last 6 years of his life Sutherland noticed even slower movements, which expanded and deepened his work. After his death in 1954 these were further studied by some of this students, in particular Rollin Becker and Ruby Day. Both taught American osteopath James S. Jealous, who today is the representative of Biodynamic Cranial Osteopathy. This treatment approach has also been adopted by some craniosacral therapy schools and so is being continuously developed further.

The various slow rhythms / tidal movements:
- about 6 – 12 cycles per minute: craniosacral rhythm;
- about 2 – 3 cycles per minute: mid-tide;
- 1 cycle per 100 seconds (about 1 cycle per 1.5 minutes): long-tide.

With a bit of practice you can listen in a more differentiated way when palpating slower movements:

The more your body relaxes and releases tensions, the better you can perceive the craniosacral rhythm with about 6 to 12 cycles per minute. This perception often happens after a pause when the craniosacral rhythm has stopped briefly (stillpoint) and then continues. With about 6 cycles per minute you can feel the unrestricted craniosacral rhythm in paired body parts for about 5 seconds as outer rotation and about 5 seconds as inner rotation. With about 10 cycles per minute it is about 3 seconds for the outer rotation, 3 seconds for the inner rotation.

If your body relaxes more deeply, for example after an endogenous (self-activated) stillpoint, you can occasionally notice even slower tidal movements. With about 3 cycles per minute (the so-called mid-tide), it takes about 10 seconds or more for the outer rotation/inhalation phase – about 2 to 4 times slower than the craniosacral rhythm.

In mid-tide the sense of structure and boundaries can dissolve. Instead it feels rather energetically flowing, as if the cells breathe. In this condition of deep relaxation there is no further activation of stillpoints or relaxation from the outside. The self-regulation already works to such an extent that activity from outside would be rather disruptive. Observe without any goals what develops further.

In deep relaxation, often after the mid-tide has been present for a while and established itself, it is possible to palpate the so-called long-tide with

1 cycle in about 100 seconds (1 cycle in about 1.5 minutes). With about 50 seconds for the outer rotation/inhalation phase and about 50 seconds for the inner rotation/exhalation phase, the long-tide is significantly slower than the mid-tide.

Sensing the long-tide when alone is easier for people who have already enjoyed several biodynamic craniosacral treatments and are experienced in meditation or deep relaxation. Often the long-tide only shows when a skilled therapist offers a safe framework and reference point.

In mid-tide as well as in long-tide it is recommended that you be present without any purpose – neutral, without judging – to marvel, to enjoy and to observe whatever wants to unfold and develop in the moment.

Palpating becomes more passive and turns into a sensitive neutral listening and observing. Even thoughts or intentions give way to the sensitive perception of these slow tidal movements.

The deeper settings and hidden secrets never show themselves with impatience and force but rather with gentle looking and observing. By going within and being still we gain insight into the core of our existence. We can marvel and feel great joy and humility when we are touched by the breath of life.

Do not judge yourself or your body or the slow tidal movements. There is no better or worse, no goal or anything else to achieve. Like the mid- and long-tide, the craniosacral rhythm is an expression of life force. All slower tidal movements give evidence of the ability of the nervous system to pulsate with certain conditions of excitement or relaxation.

Greet all rhythms as direct expression of life force, as all support self-regulation and self-healing energies. Trust your sensations and allow yourself time to listen to the various rhythms and changes in your body.

With growing experience you will receive increasingly clear and deep sensations for the various slow movements of your body. Do not force anything. If your craniosacral rhythm or slower tidal movements do not surface, follow the other body rhythms as described in the exercises on page 71. Enjoy the relaxation that becomes noticeable in the body and allows even further expansion.

Relaxing the craniosacral system

Reminders

A reminder before starting to relax the craniosacral system: Do not perform these exercises when feeling discomfort or pain, or if you have a chronic medical condition, without prior consultation with a doctor or naturopathic expert.

The self-treatments described in this book do not replace an individual craniosacral treatment with a competent craniosacral practitioner. The self-treatments excellently lend themselves to getting to know the craniosacral work and can also support and complement relaxation between individual professional treatments. Further information on what a professional craniosacral treatment comprises and what it can help with can be found on page 130–131.

If there is an exercise that you cannot do or that does not feel comfortable, just leave it aside. A reminder: For exercises lying on your back, place a rolled-up blanket beneath your knees in order to relieve tension in the torso.

The quality of touch and exact finger and hand positions

As already described in Part 2, relaxation happens not with pressure but through conscious touch inviting more space and expanse. In particular the facial and cranial bones should always be touched gently and very softly with 1 to 3 grams maximum pressure (.03 to .10 ounce).

The exact position is important as with a bit of practice you palpate via the structure the function – i.e., via the tissue the movement of the craniosacral rhythm and its qualities. The following anatomical illustrations and photos will help you with exploring and discovering the right spots.

Due to our uniqueness, the body's structure – i.e., the tissue – is different with every person. Therefore gently start feeling the structure in order to then touch exactly the right place. That is "anatomy live": in the course of this you will freshly discover your body, or rather, deepen your knowledge of it.

The more you listen to the various movements of your body with your hands, the more your sensitivity for a differentiated perception of the various slow rhythms is enhanced.

Touching activates various receptors in different depths of the tissue. Via sensory nerve messages, the soft touch is transmitted to the brain where it stimulates and activates specific areas of the brain. If a touch is light, supportive, enjoyable, the brain's feedback to the tissue is something like, "Oh, mmmm, goooood – everything okay – we surrender our resistance and stop holding fast, aaaahhh – relax further, please!" If a touch happens fast or with firm pressure, the brain most likely perceives this as an attack: immediately, automatically and instinctively the body moves into a posture of defense and protection, thus doing exactly the opposite of what we actually intended!

This is another reason that we keep reminding readers that all touch and invitations to relaxation need to be performed slowly, gently and with awareness. We want to relax the craniosacral system through loving touch.

You can notice the relaxation when the tissue under your hands starts getting wider, softer, warmer or fuller, the breathing changes or a spontaneous sigh escapes. As the tissue relaxes the cell memory can signal this with the so-called "therapeutic pulse" (strong throbbing, pulsing, prickling, release of warmth/coldness, twitching of the muscles, discharges). Keep touching the tissue until the therapeutic pulse has dissolved. How does the tissue feel after this relaxation?

Relaxing the sacrum   ca. 2 – 5 min. per exercise

lying down, possibly sitting

The sacrum is the "south pole" of the craniosacral system. Its Latin name, Os sacrum, translates into "sacred bone." A free sacrum supports the statics of the entire pelvis and its functions.

These self-treatments support and promote::
- the spine and the entire musculoskeletal system;
- the torso from sacrum upwards to the occipital bone;
- relaxation in the entire pelvic area and the lower spinal dura mater;
- a more balanced craniosacral rhythm and thereby fewer faulty positions and dysfunctions of the craniosacral system.

There are various ways of relaxing the sacrum. In the following you will learn a few simple and effective exercises.

The self-treatments below are *not recommended* with acute sciatica or lumbago, slipped disk, hip complaints, injuries of the meniscus or similar troubles. This also applies if you have had recent operations on any of these areas.

Lying on the back with knees bent / legs drawn up
Moving the sacrum slowly: Through small movements of the legs and the sacrum, numerous muscles, ligaments, strings of fascia and the connection of the sacrum with the pelvis and loin/groin area get stretched. It is particularly valuable to feel this stretch consciously and then perceive how good the relaxation feels. The new body feeling can thus be deepened.

Performing the exercises

1. Moving the sacrum

Once you lie down on your back, draw your feet up to your bottom, with both your knees bent. Release the weight of your pelvis and sacrum downward. Feel your sacrum and nestle as much of its surface as possible into the base. This results in a slight movement of the sacrum that you slowly and with pleasure continue, complementing it with slight movements originating in the hips.

Perform slight tilting movements with the sacrum: first the upper part of the sacrum moves down towards the base surface and thus the coccyx moves slightly towards the ceiling, then vice versa.

At times these movements with sacrum and hips can also be performed more actively, always though with joy and no effort. Play with the speed: alter it occasionally and in the course of this frequently allow yourself some slow movements. Finally release the whole weight of the pelvis and the sacrum to the base again. Sense into how this area now feels.

2. Positioning the sacrum further towards the feet

Briefly lift your pelvis and sacrum slightly towards the ceiling, lightly rock it towards the feet and then lay it down again on the base. Your sacrum is now positioned a few centimeters further towards the feet. Now consciously release again the weight of your sacrum, pelvis, loin/groin area, spine, entire torso and head down into the base. The new position of the sacrum lowered further towards the feet results in a slight stretch up into the torso, up to the base of the skull.

Do you feel this subtle stretch of the spine, along the spinal dura mater? Do you feel how the various muscles, ligaments and strings of fascia of pelvis, belly, chest and neck expand?

You can deepen this process through breathing consciously and letting your lower jaw drop slightly. Feel how the structures relax and how enjoyable it is when relaxation, space and expanse happen by themselves.

3. Playfully moving the pelvis

Slowly move your pelvis in all directions, including diagonally, in a way that feels good to you. This can be combined with the tilting movements of the sacrum described earlier.

Allow yourself a break in between to sense how your body now feels.

4. Moving both knees together, slightly to the right or to the left

Let both legs – slightly drawn up as they are – playfully drop to one side with their own weight. The knees remain parallel to one another and thus drift *together*, alternately to the left and to the right. This stretches the area of hips, pelvis and sacrum, as well as the area of the loins/groin up to the chest and neck, depending on how far you perform the sideward movement and how elastic the tissue is.

Let your knees topple over to the side only as far as the tissue easily accommodates. Accept the boundary. You never push the structure any further than it wants to go. At the end of the sideward movement you can stop for a few moments, consciously perceive the tension and breathe it out.

Occasionally alter direction and tempo of the movement, and allow yourself breaks to feel into your body.

5. Moving both knees away from and towards each other

Draw your legs slightly up. Now let your knees smoothly fall apart sideways and then move them back together. This stretches and revives the area of the hips, the pelvis and the sacrum. Occasionally change the distance between your knees when you move them apart. Vary the speed, down to slow motion. Every now and again feel into your body. Let your legs move only as far to the side as the tissue easily accommodates.

All of these exercises can be combined.

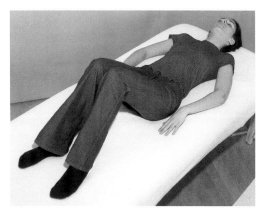 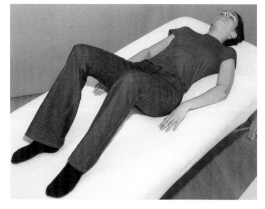

Moving drawn-up legs: relaxing sacrum, pelvis and hips

Positioning your hands flat under the sacrum: When the weight of pelvis and sacrum rests on your open hands, parts of the posterior muscles, in particular in the lateral area of the sacrum, the iliosacral joints, are relaxed.

As the pelvis is positioned slightly higher this effects a subtle stretch of the entire area of the loins/groin. In addition the spinal dura mater expands. Conscious breathing into the segment of the belly and the pelvis assists in this relaxation and gives more space.

Performing the exercise

1. Make sure you are lying comfortably. As described in the previous second exercise (p. 75), position your sacrum a bit further towards the feet and allow yourself time to notice the enjoyable stretch upwards along the torso. Trust the weight of your pelvis and sacrum to the base. Your torso, neck area and head are also invited to release tension and weight downwards. Place your extended hands, with palms facing the base, at your sides next to the pelvis.

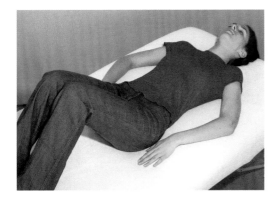
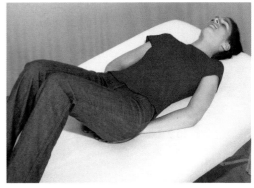

Placing flat hands under the sacrum

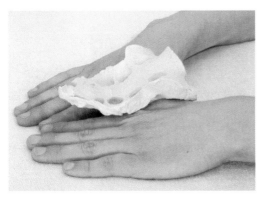

2. Now you slightly lift the pelvis, loosely position both hands under sacrum and pelvis and then again release the weight to hands and base. Does this position feel right? If not, place your hands differently, maybe a bit higher or further down, perhaps slightly more towards the middle or to the side, until it feels comfortable.

3. The first time, it is recommended not to leave the hands underneath the pelvis for too long. The hands might not be used to the weight of the pelvis. If you do this exercise on a regular basis, though, your hands will become more flexible and will relax at the same time. Instead of one minute, the hands can then remain 3 to 5 minutes under the sacrum/pelvis without feeling uncomfortable.

If the position of your hands feels fine, take your time. Again release all the weight of pelvis and sacrum. Notice the relaxation in the area of the pelvis and the loins/groin, maybe also in other body parts, and allow yourself to relax. After a while move your hands again. With loose wrists, lightly shake out your hands and fingers with all its joints.

Placing fists flat (back of hand up) or raised (thumb up) underneath the sacrum: With flat or raised fists, sacrum and pelvis are positioned considerably higher than with flat hands. Using the fists, the stretch in the pelvis and from there into the area of the loins/groin and the lower part of the spinal dura mater increases. Try out which of these positions feels most comfortable to you:

1. Flat fists:

As in the previous exercises you lie relaxed on your back with knees slightly drawn up and place your hands flat next to the pelvis, palms touching the base. Now your hands form fists that you position flat underneath the sacrum. Instead of on flat hands, as in the previous exercise, your sacrum is now placed on flat fists.

Does this position feel right? If not, slightly shift the fists until it feels comfortable or return to the open hand position of before.

2. Raised fists:

As in the previous exercises you lie relaxed with knees slightly drawn up and place your hands at your sides, palm-down next to the pelvis. Now each of your hands form a fist that is raised (thumb on top, slightly to the side). The closed palms face the sides of the pelvis. Instead of your flat fists, this time you place your raised fists underneath the area of the sacrum and pelvis. Slowly relieve the weight of the pelvis via the mounted fists to the base.

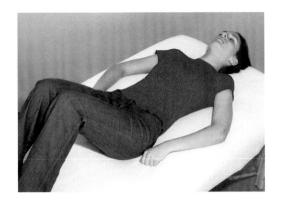

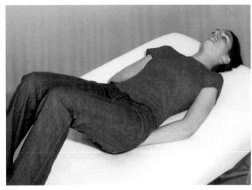

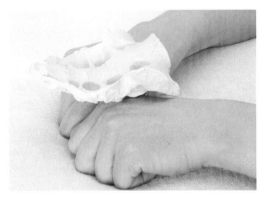

Placing flat fists
underneath the sacrum

Placing raised fists
underneath the sacrum

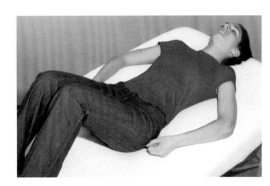

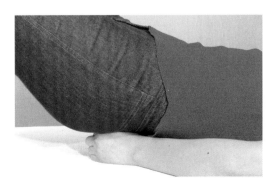

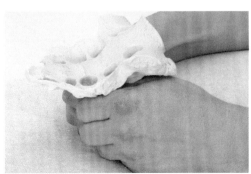

How does this feel? Is there a more fitting position of the fists, slightly higher or lower, more to the middle or to the side? Here, too, conscious breathing into the region of the belly, pelvis and sacrum assists in the relaxation.

Remove your hands; loosen the hands, fingers, wrists. Notice the local relaxation in the area of the pelvis and the loins/groin. Then relax into whole-body awareness. If the position of raised fists does not feel comfortable for either torso or fists, then simply return to the position of flat fists or hands.

Relaxing the sacrum in lateral position   ca. 2 – 5 min.

lying down

This self-treatment supports and promotes:

- parasympathetic parts of the autonomic nervous system – e.g., for encouraging:
  - digestion,
  - faster and deeper relaxation,
  - regeneration, sleep;
- strength and balance of the craniosacral rhythm;
- relaxation of the transition to the 5th lumbar vertebra, the lumbosacral joint.

Performing the exercise

1. Lie comfortably on your side and place a cushion or a folded blanket underneath your head. If you are travelling, without cushion or blanket, lift the arm on the side you are lying on and place your head on it as comfortably as possible.

2. Move the other hand – the one you are not lying on – behind towards the back and touch the sacrum in a way that feels comfortable. Drop all unnecessary tension in the shoulder. Feel your entire body and where it touches the base and your hands, and take a few breaths.

3. Your whole palm palpates the sacrum and nestles into as much of its surface as possible. You connect your hands via the clothing with the level of the skin and the level of the bones of the sacrum. It is the same "docking" and merging with the tissue that you already know from other sensing and self-treatment exercises in Part 2 of the book.

4. Listen to the tissue. When you sense movements, perceive them in a relaxed and attentive manner:

- How does it feel?
- What do you sense underneath your hands?
- How does the touch feel from the inside, from inside the sacrum?
- Do you feel a very slow tilting movement?
- Is there a bigger tilting movement in one or the other direction?
- How slow or fast is this movement?
- Is it about 3 to 6 seconds for each direction of the movement?

5. Your hand now performs a light relief/decompression on the sacrum towards the feet: Your hand is well connected with the sacrum, adjusts it lightly but steadily towards the feet without sliding.

   Here the terms "adjusting" and "decompression" do not mean pull or pressure but a clearly-intentioned, light "invitation" and a continuous pointing at the release direction with your hand. This way you allow the tissue time to release and expand by itself.

   It is less the intensity than the length of time and the continuity of this hardly-noticeable decompression that results in the relaxing effect for the whole area of the pelvis and loins/groin via the sacrum.

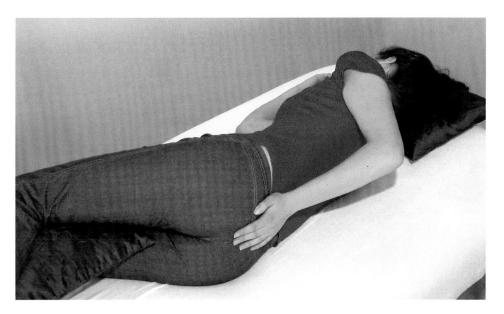

Relaxing sacrum in lateral position

6. Slowly release the steady decompression and listen without any goals. What do you perceive now underneath your hands? Do you feel differences of quality? Do you feel slow movements? If you sense the craniosacral rhythm, continue to listen through several cycles.

You can also massage the tissue on the sacrum as well as on the sides of it. This massage can then be extended to further muscles in the area of the pelvis.

Touching and relaxing the sacrum and the occipital bone
ca. 2 – 5 min.

lying on the side or on the back

Performing the exercise

1. Lie comfortably on your side, a cushion beneath your head. Move the lower of your arms under your neck towards the back of the head and place the hand with as much surface as possible on the occipital bone. At the same time the hand of the other arm touches the sacrum, in the same way as in the previous exercise.

2. Your hands feel the form and position of sacrum and occipital bone, nestling into them with as much surface contact as possible. The hands are invited to merge with both bones. Again palpate the tissue:
   - How does the sacrum feel?
   - How does the occipital bone feel?
   - What do you feel underneath your hands?
   - What happens in the dural tube between your hands?
   - Do you sense very slow, tilting movements in the area of the occipital bone and/or the sacrum?

3. Now specifically relax the spinal dura mater with a slight decompression:
   - at the sacrum towards the feet;
   - at the occipital bone towards the head;
   - at the sacrum towards the feet and at the occipital bone towards the head at the same time;
   - what do you feel before, during and after the release/decompression?

4. What do you perceive after about 3 to 5 minutes' touch and the release at these two places?
   - Is the craniosacral rhythm more pronounced, more balanced?
   - Do other body connections feel more relaxed, less restricted or more-spacious?
   - Are your sensory perceptions more intense or more differentiated?
   - Which sensory levels are more distinct: touching, listening, seeing, smelling or tasting?

For this exercise in supine position:

Lie down comfortably on your back. Position one hand across the occipital bone, covering as much surface as possible. Place the other hand with open palm flat underneath the sacrum. Try out whether it feels better with the palm up or down; this also depends on whether the surface is soft or hard.

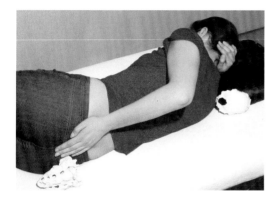

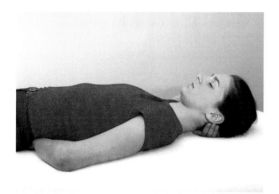

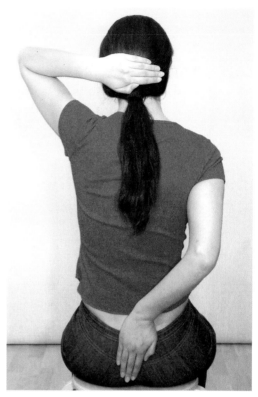

Touching sacrum and occipital bone

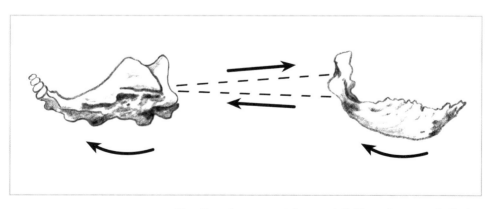

Direction of movement from occipital bone to sacrum in flexion

Relaxing the iliosacral joints
ca. 2 – 5 min.

lying down

The two iliosacral joints connect the sacrum to the iliac crests. They contribute significantly to our posture and gait. The various tissue structures of and around the iliosacral joints provide holding and stability on the one hand, and on the other hand are supposed to enable the best possible flexibility. They are frequently strained, thus often tensed up, blocked or even inflamed.

This self-treatment supports and promotes:

- the gentle stretch of the iliosacral joints and numerous ligaments and tendons, including those in deeper places;
- a less restricted sacrum;
- a stronger and more balanced craniosacral rhythm;
- elastic gait, posture and relaxation of the spine.

The previous relaxations of the sacrum constitute an excellent preparation for this, as they always relax the iliosacral joints at the same time.

Performing the exercise

In the following exercise both iliac crests are continuously invited to slide slightly inward and up.

1. Place the surfaces of both hands on your sides over the iliac crests as you did when palpating the craniosacral rhythm on the sides of the pelvis. If you only sense the skin (or the connective tissue), the following relaxation will release tissue on the superficial level alone; only when there is clear contact with the anterior superior iliac spine (Spina iliaca anterior superior) will this exercise relax the area of the iliosacral joints. Doing the latter, you feel the bony structure of the iliac crests and create a comfortable contact with your hands in that place. Deepen this by connecting both hands specifically with the bones, with as much surface contact as possible.

2. Your touch is flexible and soft, your hands listen attentively. Feel the space *between* your hands:

   - Does it want to expand?
   - Where does it feel warm or warmer?
   - Your hands listen attentively: Can you perceive body rhythms?
   - Does the tissue underneath your hands change? If so, how?

3. Now begin to move the iliac crests lightly and *continuously inward and up* with both hands simultaneously. The steady pull should be performed evenly left and right, taking from about 30 seconds to 3 minutes.

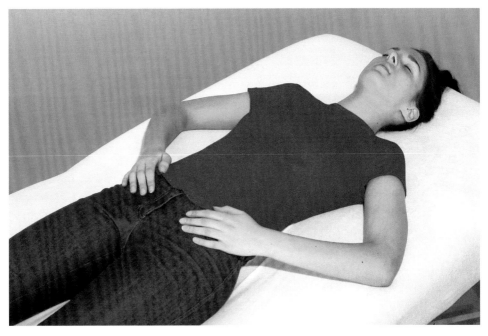

Relaxing iliosacral joints: evenly moving the iliac crests inward and up

4. When you slowly relieve the direction of the pull, your hands remain in this place and listen for a while:
    *   How does your whole pelvic area feel, your sacrum, your iliosacral joints?
    *   Do you perceive body rhythms under your hands?
    *   Is it the craniosacral rhythm? If so, what are its qualities, how slow is its movement?
    *   How do you now perceive your whole body?

At the end you can release the contact with the bony structure and continue palpating the craniosacral rhythm while touching the tissue level.

The stillpoint

Occasionally the craniosacral rhythm stops for a few seconds up to a few minutes. We call this the stillpoint. Stillpoints happen by themselves in the body, or they can be invited or, rather, activated from the outside.

Stillpoints support the craniosacral system and the regeneration of the entire body, which rests for a few minutes in the calmness of its center. During a stillpoint the entire craniosacral system harmonizes itself from the inside. During and after a stillpoint the whole rhythm of the breath often changes and a comfortable relaxation unfurls or deepens.

Stillpoints support:
- the parasympathetic nervous system, to the following effect:
  - relaxation and balance of the autonomic nervous system are improved;
  - the tonus of the connective tissue is decreased;
  - the whole musculoskeletal system, including the spine and the base of the skull, is being relaxed;
- the homeostasis – i.e., the maintenance of inner balance
- letting go on the physical, emotional, mental, soul and spiritual levels.

Stillpoints act as:
- generally relaxing, and also effective as a help in going to sleep;
- centering and strengthening – e.g., after conditions of exhaustion.

After the stillpoint:
- The craniosacral rhythm often starts up more strongly than before.
- The brain and the area around the medulla are purified and nourished by fresh cerebrospinal fluid.
- The craniosacral rhythm is often more balanced and can be noticed more distinctly.

Contraindications for stillpoints activated from the outside include:
- acute injuries/fractures on the head
- suspected cerebral hemorrhage, vascular dilatation or swelling of the meninges
- cerebral aneurysm
- stroke
- meningitis, borreliosis (Lyme Disease)

- fresh/acute whiplash; concussion, impact
- multiple sclerosis*, epilepsy *
- pregnancy in the 1st to the 3rd and the 7th to the 9th month*

The starred items (*) are listed as a measure of precaution. Please also note the general contraindications on page 23.

Activating the stillpoint on the pelvis   ca. 5 – 15 min.

lying down, possibly sitting

Performing the exercise

Everywhere that you can perceive the craniosacral rhythm on the exterior of the body as outer and inner rotation (OIR), you use the following OIR technique:

1. Lie on your back and place your hands on the sides of your pelvis, as in the iliosacral joint relaxation or when palpating the body rhythms (see pages 70–72 and 84–85. If you are sitting, touch your thighs close to the pelvis. Palpate the craniosacral rhythm in the outer and inner rotation and notice its qualities.

2. After several cycles follow with both hands (evenly) the inner rotation up to its innermost point, pause there and thus prevent the outer rotation. Subsequently the stillpoint arrives, sometimes immediately, sometimes after about half a minute to a minute. The previously-felt surge outward, into the outer rotation, decreases and falls away.

   Or:

   If you feel the craniosacral rhythm in its inner and outer rotation, you can activate the stillpoint more gently than before. You do not continuously hold the iliac crests in their innermost point of the inner rotation but take the craniosacral rhythm gently to the stillpoint by continuously slowing down and slightly restraining the outer rotation while you keep going in the inner rotation. This approach may take a bit longer and it assumes you can palpate/sense the craniosacral rhythm.

3. Stillpoint. What do you feel during the stillpoint between your hands, in your body? Perhaps fine adjustments of the body itself, even a twitching? When the calmness of the stillpoint arrives, your hands can become soft. You then no longer hold the exterior of the body in inner rotation; your hands touch only gently and listen.

   When the craniosacral rhythm with its about 6 to 12 cycles rests in a stillpoint, sometimes even slower movements can be noticed in this stillness (see pages 70–72).

Coming to know stillpoints, feeling the mid-tide or long-tide and experiencing the breath of life is always new and unique. Stillpoints will be individually experienced very differently – for example:

- with a deep outbreath or yawning;
- as enormous expansion;
- as deep peace;
- as dynamic stillness;
- as relaxation in the deepest ocean of the body or the universe;
- as the coming together of body, mind and soul.

4. When the craniosacral rhythm starts again – usually with a long outer rotation – palpate its movements for several cycles:
   - Are there differences compared to before? If so, what are they?
   - Have the qualities of the craniosacral rhythm changed after the stillpoint? If so, how?

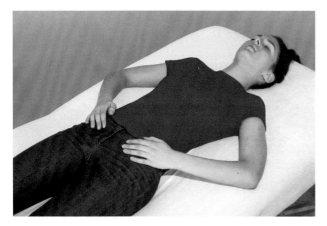

Activating stillpoint
on the pelvis

Activating the stillpoint on the occipital bone (CV4, compression of ventricle 4)   ca. 5 – 10 min.

lying down

At the cranium the stillpoint can be most easily activated on the occipital bone. The pressure effected here through the head's own weight is transmitted to the intracranial system and it influences the fourth cerebral ventricle. This ventricle is gently and continuously compressed so that after a given time a stillpoint sets in.

Note the contraindications on page 23 and page 86!

Performing the exercise

Get two soft beanbags from a toy or sports shop. Take a sock and place them inside, all the way into the toe. Tie the sock in a knot, so that the beanbags touch; they are supposed to lie right next to each other so that later on, with the weight of the head on them, they do not move apart. Now, when lying on your back, instead of a cushion place the two beanbags tied into that sock at the height of your occipital bone. Position the beanbags about 2 centimeters (1 inch) above the bottom edge of the occipital bone. It is important to place them not too low (not right at the edge of the cranium) and not too high (not at the lambdoid suture close to the parietal bones). Your head can lie relaxed on this for about 5 minutes. If you feel like it – definitely after 10 to 15 minutes, though – the sock with the beanbags can be put aside. Sense into how you now feel. Which body parts have relaxed particularly well?

This exercise is not for everybody, and the beanbags may not always feel comfortable. If this is the case, activate the stillpoint on the sides of the pelvis or on the thighs.

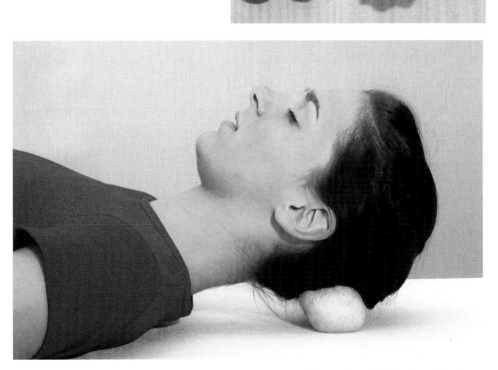

Activating stillpoint in occipital bone

Relaxing the connective tissue ca. 3 – 5 min. per position

sitting, lying down, possibly standing

Healthy exercise, combined with several professional craniosacral treatments and various other body therapies, relaxes the transverse connective tissue. Regular self-treatments support this beautifully. When transverse structures relax, this has a relieving effect on the longitudinal connective tissue structures that are interwoven with them.

The connective tissue of our body is a great matrix. When it is mostly permeable, it connects instead of separating and supports the body, in particular the musculoskeletal system and the organs, in all its functions.

This self-treatment supports and promotes:

- the pelvic floor, the diaphragm, the shoulder/neck area and the base of the skull;
- stability, strength, flexibility and mobility of the body;
- the mutual exchange of information between segments and the brain;
- the vessels, thus improving blood supply and detoxification;
- the free course of the vagus nerve, which improves vegetative functions; this in turn enhances the digestion, functions of the heart and breath, the communication of "head brain" and "belly brain";
- the free, spontaneous expression of our life force and joy of life.

The connective tissue release technique applied here is easy and effective. You perform it similarly as in the self-treatment "Perceiving, relaxing and connecting body segments" in Part 2 (pages 51–59). If you learned that one, you can consider the following exercise an extension of it. The difference is that here it particularly addresses and relaxes those areas of the body with a lot of transverse connective tissue.

Performing the exercise (for all positions)

1. With loose hands gently touch the chosen body segment, or two segments. The hands and fingers should touch as much surface area as possible – just as if your hand were being modelled by the underlying perceivable structure – without tension in hands, fingers or wrists. Occasionally close your eyes in order to direct the attention more towards the inner and perceive the relaxation from the inside, as well.

2. The surfaces of your hands and fingers can connect with the area, as if merging with it. Let your sensory awareness work for you: numerous receptors in your hands receive with increasing practice various pieces of information – e.g., about the mobility or warmth/coldness of the touched structure, on its surface as well as in its depth.

3. With clear, soft and space-giving contact with the surfaces of the connected fingers and hands you feel into the depth of the tissue:
   - How does this area feel?
   - Does anything change when you breathe into this segment from the inside a few times?
   - What do you feel underneath your hands?
   - How does this touch feel from the inside?

4. You can slowly, slightly increase the intensity of the touch of hands and fingers and thus connect more accurately with deeper tissue. You do not exercise any invading pressure, as this often provokes the structure to (natural) protective reactions such as contracting. The tension is not being broken with manually invasive techniques but softened, relieved with "awareness through touch." Accept the tension as a natural border and wait with conscious and harmonious touch until the tissue beneath your hands relaxes by itself.

Implementation:
The following positions demonstrate a few of the numerous possible combinations. You can choose intuitively or you can relax the transverse connective tissue from the bottom to the top. Occasionally close your eyes in order to perceive the relaxation from the inside.

Pelvic area:
One open-palmed hand touches across the pelvic area. The small fingers touch the loins/groin or are placed as closely as possible to the loin area.

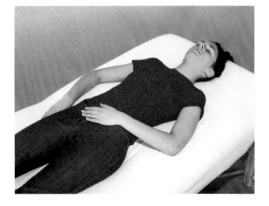

Relaxing
pelvic area

Diaphragm:
The open palm of one hand touches the lower rib arch and thus makes contact with the transition from belly to ribcage and the area of the diaphragm underneath.

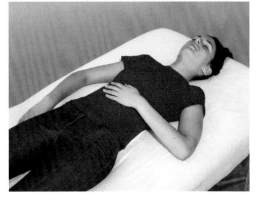

Relaxing
diaphragm

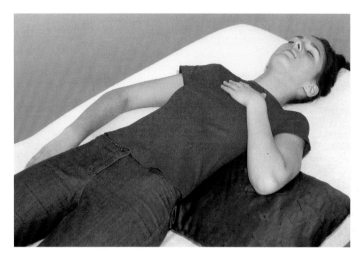

Upper entry to the ribcage: One hand touches and relaxes the entry to the upper ribcage. Thumb and index finger touch the collarbones while hand and fingers touch the ribcage with as much surface as possible.

Relaxing upper entry to ribcage

Touching the hyoid:
As shown on the photos below, for this exercise you specifically touch the hyoid bone (Os hyoideum) on the throat. The hyoid is the only bone in the body that is not directly connected to others. Many muscles, ligaments and sinews are attached to it, leading upwards to the floor of the mouth, the tongue, the lower jaw and the styloid process of the temporal bone (Os temporale), downwards to the larynx, the sternum, the collarbones and the shoulder blades.

The relaxed hyoid assists with:
- language and voice development;
- a relaxed floor of the mouth;
- the connection to the styloid process of the temporal bone;
- the thyroid function.

Implementation
You find the hyoid by gently placing the surface of the thumb and index finger of one hand a few centimeters apart, clearly above the larynx and directly underneath the floor of the mouth. Allow yourself time so that the surfaces of your fingers can gently and slowly connect with the tissue, without pressure. Find out whether you are really touching the hyoid: move your tongue a few times up to the palate and back to the floor of the mouth, or swallow several times. By doing this the hyoid bone is moved upwards and downwards and is easier to feel with thumb and index finger.

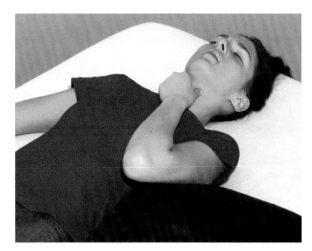

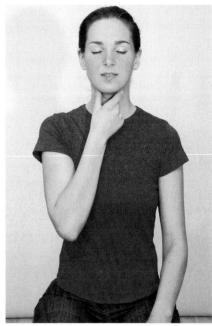

Touching hyoid and
relaxing the throat area

Relaxing the base of the skull:
Place both hands with open palms across the occipital bone (from behind).
The fingers are slightly spread and intertwined. Both thumbs are positioned
at the edge of the skull of the occipital bone and touch it clearly, gently and
without pressure. You palpate and touch the tissue with both thumbs – for
example, the onset of the muscles at the edge of the occiput, as described
before. You listen, palpate, invite spaciousness and expanse and allow yourself some time. This relaxes the base of the skull that is at the same level.

How does the structure feel underneath your hands?
- Can you feel the craniosacral rhythm?
- What happens between your hands, in the area of the atlanto-occipi-
tal joint?
- Do the onsets of the muscles become softer, wider, more elastic?

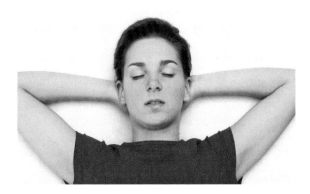

Relaxing the base
of the skull

Relaxing the connective tissue
– combination

ca. 3 – 5 min. per position

sitting, lying down, possibly standing

Performing the exercise (see page 90)

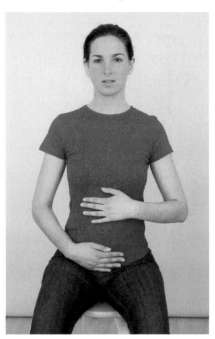

Relaxing pelvic and diaphragm areas

Pelvis and diaphragm:
One hand touches transverse connective tissue in the pelvic area. The small fingers touch the loins/groin or are placed as closely as possible to the loin area. The whole surface of the other hand touches the lower costal arch, makes contact with the diaphragm and relaxes this area. If position and touch feel right, you can close your eyes and keep your attention with your sensory awareness.

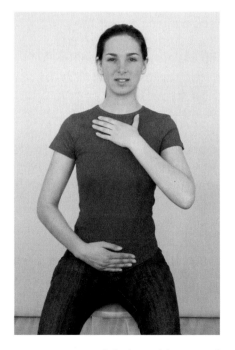

Relaxing pelvic area and
upper entry to ribcage

Pelvis and upper ribcage:
One hand continues to touch the pelvic area. The other hand touches and relaxes the area around the upper entry of the ribcage. Thumb and index finger touch the collarbones; the fingers and hands touch with as much surface as possible.

Further possibilities: With the lower hand remaining in the pelvic area, the upper hand now touches the hyoid and relaxes the area of the throat. Further up this hand can also extensively touch and relax the upper area of the neck and the transition to the occipital bone, and thus the structure of the base of the skull at the same level.

Diaphragm and upper entry to the ribcage:
One hand touches the lower costal arch extensively, making contact with the area of the diaphragm and thus relaxing the transition from belly to ribcage. The other hand touches and relaxes the upper entry to the ribcage. Thumb and index finger touch the collarbones; the fingers and hands touch with as much surface as possible.

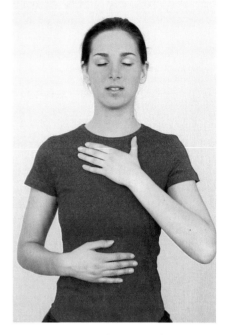

Relaxing diaphragm area
and upper entry to ribcage

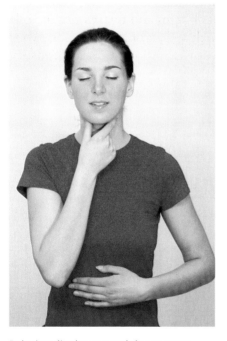

Relaxing diaphragm and throat areas

Diaphragm and throat:
The hand positioned in the area of the diaphragm can remain there while the other hand touches the hyoid and relaxes the area of the throat.

Subsequently, the hand touching the hyoid contacts with as much surface as possible the upper neck area and the transition to the occipital bone. It relaxes the atlanto-occipital joint and the base of the skull while the other hand rests in the area of the diaphragm.

Neck and base of the skull:
One hand touches extensively the upper neck area from behind, across. The little finger touches the edge of the occipital bone. The whole hand makes contact with the upper neck area. The other hand touches across the occipital bone and merges with its form. The thumb of this hand can touch the little finger of the other hand. If the upper neck area and the transition to the occipital bone relax, the base of the skull that sits at the same level relaxes too.

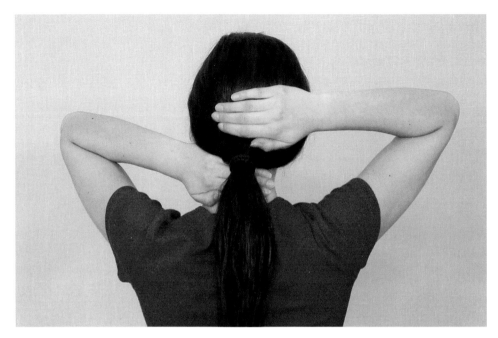

Relaxing neck area and base of skull

What does the structure feel like underneath one hand? What do you feel beneath the other? Can you feel the craniosacral rhythm as more pronounced with the one hand on the occipital bone, the more the neck area relaxes beneath the other hand? What happens between your hands, in the area of the atlanto-occipital joint?

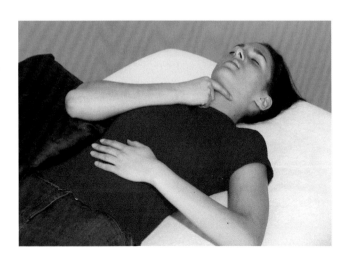

Relaxing diaphragm
and throat areas

Diaphragm and throat:
One hand touches and relaxes the area of the diaphragm; the other hand contacts the hyoid and relaxes the throat area.

Upper entry to the ribcage and throat:
One hand touches the upper entry to the ribcage; the other hand contacts the hyoid and relaxes the throat area.

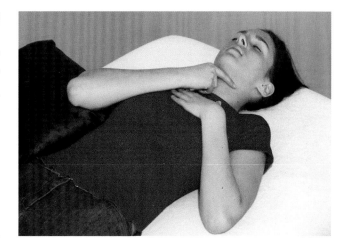

Relaxing upper entry to ribcage and throat areas

Relaxing the connective tissue with light fascia gliding

ca. 2 – 5 min. per position

lying down

"Fascia gliding" serves as another way of relaxing connective tissue and muscles. Fascia are mantles of individual organs, muscles or groups of muscles that consist of collagen fibres and elastic networks. They sheathe the musculature everywhere in the area of the face, neck, torso and extremities and serve as an organic sheath under the skin. You can apply fascia gliding anywhere on your body.

Performing the exercise

1. One or two hands connect through the clothes, initially with the layer of the skin and then gently with the layers of connective tissue underneath. As your hand connects with the structure, you move it slightly vertically upwards or downwards and then horizontally to the left or the right, *without sliding on the surface*. Note the resistance of the skin with this gentle moving and shifting of the layers of the connective tissue. You pull the skin and the layers of the connective tissue and fascia underneath only as far as the free tissue allows without resistance. If you feel a resistance in the tissue while moving it, accept this stop as a natural boundary and keep your hand at this place. Keep your attention in this place and for a few moments breathe into this area from the inside.

2. As a result, the tissue releases (often through the warmth and gentleness of the touch), allowing you to continue the slight pull of the tissue

in the same direction as before. With the next stop, when your hands notice a renewed resistance of the tissue, you repeat as before. You can then choose whether to move and relax the tissue in the opposite direction – that is, horizontally instead of vertically. You can also continue to follow the free or freed-up directions of the tissue.

3. Once fascia gliding releases the tissue underneath your hands, it generally gets softer. Then you can slowly reconnect with the deeper layers of the tissue that still hold fast, through somewhat more intense touch. If your hand has clear contact with the deeper layers of the tissue, you can continue sliding the fascia and contacting and relaxing deeper structures again and again.

Or:

Instead of connecting your hands with the depth of the tissue, you can touch the surface only lightly but extensively and let the tissue underneath your hands expand.

During the fascia gliding you can close your eyes and direct your attention to your hands, to the touched and releasing tissue, as well as to your holistic body awareness. Fascia gliding happens without any application of pressure; it is more of a gliding or "surfing" on the surface of the skin or muscles.

With some practice you can relax the coverings around the organs and the organs themselves through fascia gliding combined with other self-treatments. Craniosacral therapy calls this visceral treatment; osteopathy calls it visceral manipulation. Performed by a therapist this treatment is recommended for improving the posture and all body functions. The therapist uses it for relaxing the tissue – for example, before operations. Before, during and after a pregnancy the therapist supports the big changes in the body of the mother through visceral treatment.

Fascia gliding is often used in combination with relaxing the segments and the transverse connective tissue.

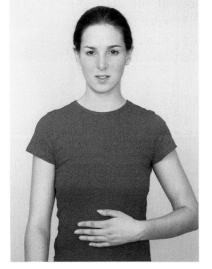

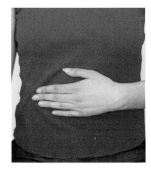

Fascia gliding: without sliding the hand over the surface, the tissue is being moved slightly

Relaxing the head / cranial bones

Before relaxing at the head

Before demonstrating gentle relaxations at the head, here is another reminder about contraindications. As a precaution do not perform any self-treatment at the head if any one of the following applies, or shortly thereafter: meningitis, injuries/fractures to the head, concussion, whiplash, stroke, illnesses of the nervous system (multiple sclerosis, epilepsy), longer spells of feeling unwell, pressure in the head or headaches/migraines.

The self-treatments serve as preventative health care and relaxation; they are not for treating ailments or illnesses. If you feel unwell for a longer stretch of time, check the causes with a doctor or alternative practitioner, and possibly visit a professional craniosacral practitioner afterwards.

It is suggested that beginners in craniosacral self-treatment initially perform the exercises in the order listed here. You first relax the base of the skull (attached to which are numerous muscles, running from the torso upwards), then feel for the cranial sutures and subsequently find more easily the individual cranial bones, where you palpate the quality characteristics of the craniosacral rhythm (see page 69).

For integrating the relaxations in the area of the head, I recommend about 2 to 3 touches/positions in the torso, pelvis and sacrum areas.

Even just listening to the craniosacral rhythm is an exciting and relaxing exercise, a meditative journey with the tidal rhythms of our nervous system. Through differentiated listening to the qualities (movements) of the craniosacral rhythm, we receive continuous clues about free or sluggish body areas. Every single structure – e.g., a cranial bone – has it own motility that depends on the mobility of the entire system. If a structure is relaxed, its improved motility will subsequently improve overall mobility. Our body possesses immense powers of self-regulation that balance the changes of motility and mobility. If the self-regulation is not sufficient, I recommend about 6 to 12 supportive treatments with a professional craniosacral practitioner.

Listen accurately at the structure to the slow movements of the craniosacral rhythm and listen differentially to its qualities: What is the speed, the spaciousness of the movement, its strength? Are there differences between left and right on the paired bones of the cranium?

After performing the self-palpation at the cranial bones you will also be able to perform some easy relaxations of the craniosacral system. You palpate again and compare the craniosacral rhythm with the movements before the self-relaxation. Thus you have a "before – after" comparison and can continue the same self-treatment or proceed with other exercises, or combine them.

The more often you do the self-treatments in this part of the book, the more confidence you will gain, both with the exact positions and with the differentiated perception of the slow tidal movements of your body. The more familiar you are with these exercises, the less you have to stick to this order and the more you decide intuitively which exercise you perform for how long and how you combine the exercises.

Relaxing the base of the skull and the occipital bone

ca. 5 min.

lying down, sitting

This self-treatment enhances:
- spaciousness and expansion in the area of the atlanto-occipital joint;
- the relaxation of the base of the skull and the area of the upper neck;
- the indirect relaxation of the temporomandibular joint.

Performing the exercise

In the exercise "Relaxing the connective tissue" (see page 93), you place both hands simultaneously on the occipital bone and with both thumbs on the edge of the occipital bone you relax the tissue in the area of the atlanto-occipital joint and at the base of the skull. The following exercise helps you to address and relax the base of the skull and the occipital bone even more directly.

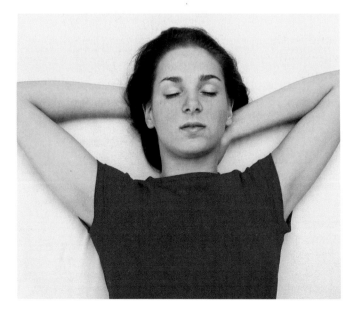

Relaxing base of skull and occipital bone

1. Place one hand across the occipital bone, so that the thumb directly touches its lower edge. The other hand extensively touches the area of the upper neck from behind, transversely. The edge of the little finger touches the edge of the occipital bone, possibly even slightly touching the thumb of the other hand. The lower hand contacts the area of the upper neck with as much surface as possible. You make clear contact, listen, feel, invite spaciousness and expansion and thus relax the base of the skull that lies horizontally between your hands.

   • What does the structure feel like beneath your hands?
   • Can you feel the craniosacral rhythm at the occipital bone?
   • What happens between your hands, in the area of the transition from the first cervical to the occipital condyles, the atlanto-occipital joint?

2. Once the tissue has started releasing, you can also put your hand on the occipital bone and perform a gentle, barely-imagined decompression towards the top of the head. This hand slides minimally, about 1 to 2 millimeters (3/4 of an inch) towards the top of the head. The result of this is an initially hardly-discernible stretch in the whole area of the neck that also affects the shoulders and the upper area of the spinal dura mater/dural tube.

This gentle release of pressure/decompression is not active, noticeable pull (traction), but a clear invitation indicating a direction, which is as subtle as the flap of a butterfly's wings.

Instead of being fast, brief and with force, this gentle decompression happens slowly, lightly and steadily for about 30 seconds up to 3 minutes.

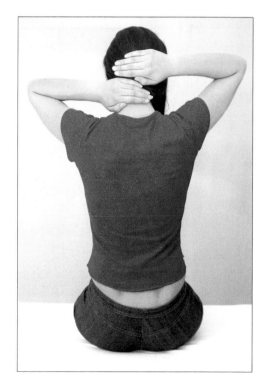

Relaxing base of skull
and occipital bone

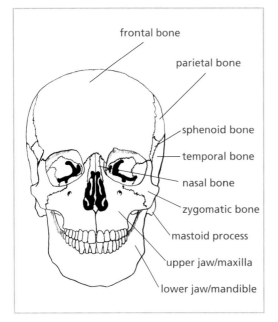

Cranial bones from the front

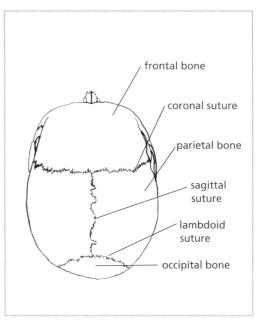

Cranial bones and cranial sutures from above

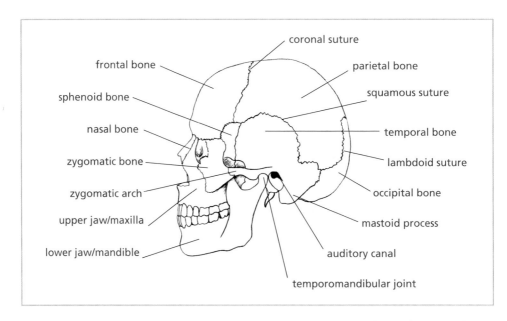

Cranial bones and cranial sutures sideways

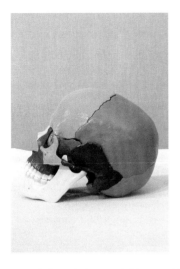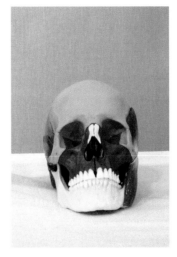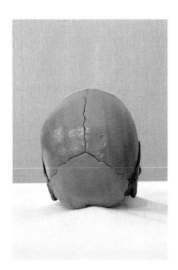

From left to right: cranial bones sideways, front and back

Feeling and relaxing the cranial sutures ca. 2 min. per position

lying down, sitting

With the following exercise you feel, touch and relax individual cranial sutures. This facilitates accurate listening to the craniosacral rhythm on various cranial bones in subsequent exercises. Important here is the exact touch and the warmth of your fingertips (meaning the whole surface of the upper phalanx which enables a particularly sensitive touch). Equally essential is your intention and invitation to allow spaciousness and expansion underneath your hands, as all this is being transferred to the brain by numerous receptors in the sutures and elsewhere.

This self-treatment supports and promotes:
- the expansion of the cranial sutures;
- the relaxation of the meninges and the intracranial membranes;
- an unrestricted, balanced craniosacral rhythm.

As described in the chapters "The craniosacral system" (page 11) and "The craniosacral rhythm" (page 67), our cranial sutures are not solidly grown together. The "cranial breathing" in fact depends on the flexibility of all structures of the craniosacral system. Through the birth process or falls, the cranial sutures can, however, be partly compressed, wedged, or very narrow and compact.

The illustrations with the names of the cranial bones and sutures, along with the color photos, facilitate finding the structure when feeling for it. I recommend looking at these and becoming familiar with the details.

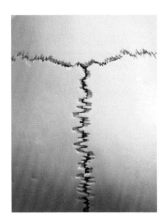

Coronal and sagittal sutures with bregma

While photos and descriptions help, only you can discover how this information affects your body, as every person is unique. When you compare the right-left side of paired body structures, not one is absolutely identical to the other; even the arching form and the course of the sutures can vary slightly.

At least as important as the knowledge of the anatomy is to connect it with the practice of palpating. You can read as much as you like; in the end, having the experience is what counts. You need to investigate, feel and through listening and following support the movement and thus the self-regulation. Thus these self-help exercises develop into discovery journeys where we can experience and learn many new things from and with our body. This can happen without stress, in relaxed slowness.

Performing the exercise

With very light touch of your fingertips, feel the following cranial sutures underneath the scalp. They can stand out through a more or less slight ridge or dimple or a change of form. Again: touch, contact, invite spaciousness and expansion.

The coronal suture (Sutura coronalis): Connects frontal bone and parietal bones. You place your fingertips on the upper area of the forehead where the coronal suture can usually be palpated, slightly beyond the hairline.

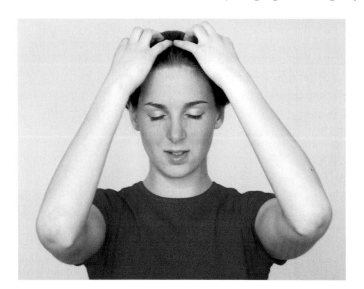

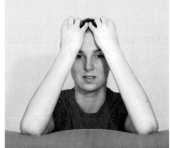

Elbows propped up: feeling and relaxing coronal suture

Palpating and relaxing coronal suture

The sagittal suture (Sutura sagittalis): Connects the pair of parietal bones. The fingernails of both hands touch slightly. With your fingertips feel the sagittal suture on the highest point on the head's midline. This leads towards the front to the bregma (the connection to the frontal bone) and towards the back to the lambdoid point (the connection to the occipital bone). Feel the sagittal suture along its course.

The squamous suture (Sutura squamosa): Connects the temporal bones, positioned sideways on the head, with the parietal bones. Your fingertips touch the scalp above the ears and feel for the structure. Occasionally you palpate a bit higher and deeper, in order to find the slightly-overlapping squamous suture.

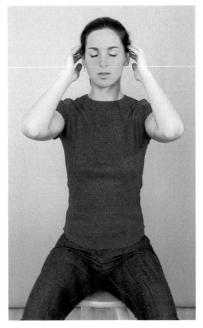

Feeling and relaxing the squamous suture

Gently massaging the cranial sutures: If your fingertips have listened for some time and if you perceive, for example, spaciousness, expansion, warmth, you can expand the self-treatment by lightly massaging the sutures with slow and gentle circling movements. This happens not in the depth of the sutures or with pressure but on the surface and much more slowly and gently than when you wash your hair.

Touching the cranial bones and listening to their movements
ca. 5 min. per position

lying down, sitting

Having already felt the cranial sutures on your head in the previous exercise, it is easy now to find and accurately touch the individual cranial bones. The illustrations and photos on pages 102–103 assist you in becoming familiar with the possibly new concepts and terms and to touch the right spots. You can follow the order listed or determine it yourself intuitively.

Implementation
As already described in Parts 1 and 2 of this book, when sitting make sure you are grounded and centered, your breath flowing easily and the area of the shoulder and neck as loose as possible. Your lower jaw can drop slightly. You do not need to strain yourself.

Even your intention of being receptive to connecting with the various levels (hair, scalp, head bones, meninges, cerebrospinal fluid), creates openness for resonance. Our level of sensory awareness is being trained and expanded; our nervous system becomes sensitized for new impressions. All this happens without effort but with ease. Let the rhythm come to you!

The ability to palpate and listen more deeply is supported by:

- the anatomically exact finger position and the soft, gentle contact;
- your mental attitude: equanimity instead of concentration;
- the duration (whether you listen, e.g., for 3 minutes or only for 30 seconds in one spot);
- the regularity of palpating: daily, weekly, more often.

Feel the structure of each cranial bone and the sutures that you have come to know (as connection to the neighboring structure) in the previous exercise, one at a time. This time you touch *not* the cranial sutures but the surface of the cranial bones. As preparation for this I recommend the previous exercise and palpating the body rhythms. Craniosacral treatment that you may have received from a professional practitioner will also facilitate self-palpating.

Performing the exercise

1. Touching the chosen cranial bones happens with much surface of the fingers, slowly and gently. Occasionally close your eyes in order to perceive the relaxation from the inside. With as much surface as possible and without touching the cranial sutures or other cranial bones, your fingers at the cranium connect with:

   • hair;

   • the scalp;

   • the bone level.

   Allow yourself time until you are clearly connected to the level of the bones. What do you perceive here? What do you feel in your head, what in your body?

2. Now greet the meninges, positioned behind the bone. Following on from the bone level, connect with this connective tissue, the meninges. Bones have a firmer substance than the meninges, which possess a certain firmness but are, compared to the bones, more malleable, more elastic, softer, more flexible.

3. Also greet the cerebrospinal fluid and open your awareness to its flowing in and around the brain. Compared to the level of the bones and meninges, this flowing feels even finer and subtler. The extended listening and connectedness to all these structures helps everything to be in resonance so that the cranial breathing can show up more easily. Often you can touch even more lightly: let your cranium breathe freely and listen to the slow tidal movements of the craniosacral rhythm.

4. Differentiate between the named qualities of the craniosacral rhythm (see page 69) or slower rhythms. You can newly perceive them after the following relaxations at the cranium (or after a stillpoint that you activate), as a comparison. Should you palpate the mid-tide (2 to 3 cycles per minute), continue to listen without changing anything. Let yourself be surprised!

5. Consciously leave that spot and mindfully release the touch. Take a few deep breaths and open your eyes.

Do not be narrow, firm or fixed: every now and again check the intensity of the touch and continuously adjust it, in particular when a relaxation in the tissue or a stillpoint occurs.

> You really listen and palpate to the ability of local areas and the entire organism to adjust themselves. Each time, you accept when the tissue rests. You do not interfere with the (natural) self-regulation but support it through your soft touch. Allow the structure the time it needs in order to trust your inviting touch and let go. Our subconsciousness and the wisdom of the body know more than we realize. Less is often more.

Touching the frontal bone   ca. 3 – 5 min.

sitting, lying down

Exact position, gentle touch: move your hands towards the forehead and touch your frontal bone with as much surface of both hands' fingers as possible. The touch happens slowly, clearly and gently. As a beginner you feel the coronal suture above and clearly place your fingertips against it or below. The little fingers can touch. The index fingers are positioned on the frontal bone, not sideways on the head. This ensures that you do not palpate too far behind (on the parietal bones) or too far to the side (on the temporal bones). The thumbs are not on the head but can touch the index

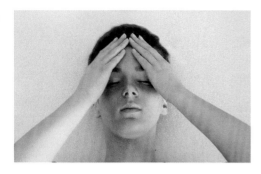

fingers without being involved or can have a slight distance from the head. The finger pads touch the eyebrows and connect softly with the lower edge of the forehead. Continue as previously described, points 1 to 5 (see pages 106–107).

Touching frontal bone and listening to craniosacral rhythm, lying down (see also photos on p. 66)

Touching and relaxing the parietal bones   ca. 5 min.

sitting, lying down

Touching the parietal bones

Exact position, gentle touch: you bring both hands sideways to your pair of parietal bones and touch these with as much surface of your fingers as possible. The touch happens slowly, clearly and gently. As a beginner, feel the coronal suture running along the upper edge of the frontal bone, and place

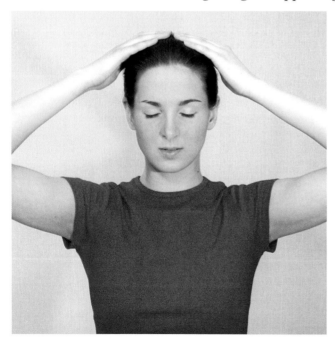

the tips of your little fingers clearly above, about 1 centimeter (less than ½ inch) behind, and to the side of the sagittal suture. The other fingertips and surfaces touch the parietal bones. The sides of the head remain free; you are not constricted by the balls of the thumbs or the heels of the hand. They do not touch the coronal suture and do not confine the squamous suture laterally. The thumbs are not involved.

Continue as previously described, points 1 to 5 (see pages 106–107).

Sitting: touching parietal bones and listening to craniosacral rhythm

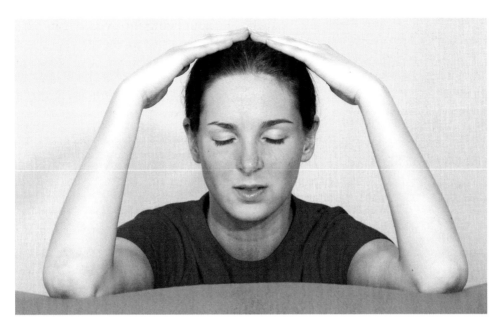

Elbows propped up: touching parietal bones and listening to craniosacral rhythm

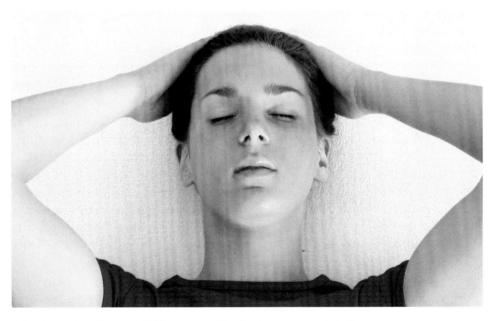

Lying down: touching parietal bones and listening to craniosacral rhythm

Relaxing the parietal bones

This self-treatment enhances:
- the flexibility of the Falx cerebri and other intracranial membranes;
- the draining of the cerebrospinal fluid, and thus better purification of the brain;
- the connection and the balance of the cerebral hemispheres;
- the ability to learn and concentrate;
- the blood circulation in the brain;
- stronger arterial and venous vessels, thus prevention of stroke;
- less restricted, more balanced craniosacral rhythm.

The relaxation of the parietal bones can be supported by:
- lightly smoothing out the temporal muscles upwards and massaging them (Exercise page 39);
- feeling for and relaxing the squamous suture (Exercise page 105).

These exercises are recommended as preparation for, as well as combined with, the exercises that follow.

Performing the exercise

After touching and listening to the parietal bones, as previously described from points 1 to 4 (pages 106-107), you have probably received an impression of the craniosacral rhythm. Now, with your intention directed towards the top of the head, invite the parietal bones to relax.

1. First, feel the squamous suture and the coronal suture (see pages 104, 105). Then place the balls of your thumbs and the heels of your hands (or fingertips) sideways with much surface on the upper end of the parietal bones, without compressing any sutures. The heels of your hands (or fingertips) leave the coronal suture untouched, and the balls of your thumbs do not contact the lambdoid suture.

2. When position and quality of touch on the paired parietal bones are congruent, you effect a gentle, barely-imagined decompression of the parietal bones towards the top of the head. This relaxes sutures, meninges and the Falx cerebri. The hands slide minimally, but steadily, about 1 to 2 millimeters (3/4 of an inch) in the cranial direction, without altering the touch of balls of the thumbs and heels of the hands (or fingertips). This gentle decompression results in a scarcely active or noticeable pull measurable in grams; primarily it brings a clear invitation in

the cranial direction. As mentioned before, this invitation is as subtle as the flap of a butterfly's wings.

Rather than being fast, brief and forceful, this decompression happens slowly, lightly and steadily over a period of 30 seconds up to 3 minutes. Afterwards you palpate whether the craniosacral rhythm on the parietal bones arises and is more pronounced and balanced, and compare before and after.

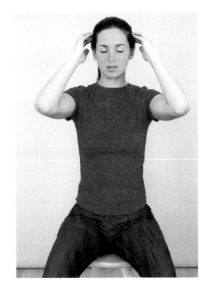

Relaxing parietal bones
with fingertips

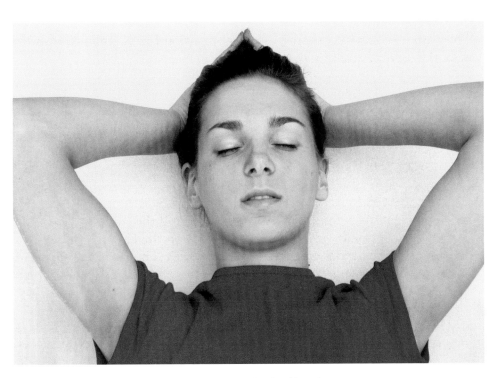

Relaxing parietal bones with balls of thumbs and heels of hands

Harmonizing Your Craniosacral System

Relaxing the temporal bones ca. 5 min.

In outer rotation the craniosacral rhythm widens the pair of temporal bones (Ossa temporalia) in the area of the squamous suture; these simultaneously rotate slightly in the direction of the facial bones. In inner rotation the temporal bones rotate in the direction of the occipital bone.

There are various reasons why these movements can be palpated not at all or only in a limited way:

- too much tension in the chewing muscles and in the area of the throat, shoulders, upper thorax, neck;
- dysfunction on the base of the skull;
- compression of different sutures of the temporal bone;
- tensions on the tentorium cerebelli and other membranes;
- imbalance at the fluid level, especially lateral movements/fluctuation
- external trauma.

Through the exercises from Parts 2 and 3 you have already relaxed structures directly connected to the temporal bones – for example, the masseter, the muscles in the area of the occipital bone, shoulders and neck, the base of the skull as well as the ribcage and neck segment.

Listening to the craniosacral rhythm at the temporal bones

With all fingertips, feel the squamous suture and then clearly place the fingertips about 1 centimeter (less than ½ inch) closer to the ear to palpate the movements of the temporal bones there. Instead of the squamous

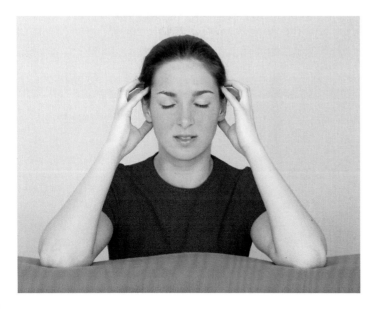

Elbows propped up:
listening to craniosacral rhythm
on temporal bones

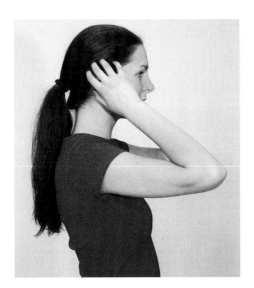
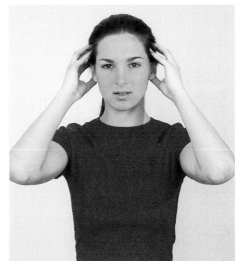
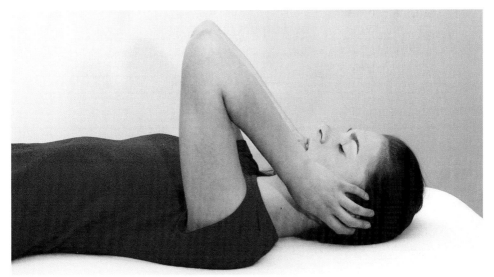

Sitting, lying: listening to craniosacral rhythm on temporal bones

suture the thumbs feel for the mastoid process behind the earlobe and are placed there. Your fingertips again connect with hair, scalp, the level of the bones and you also tune into the level of the meninges and the cerebrospinal fluid. Listen to the qualities of the craniosacral rhythm: Can you, for example, palpate the movement on the left and on the right in the same way, or differently?

Further perform the exercise as in points 1 to 5 on pages 106–107.

Relaxing the temporal bones with gentle earpull

sitting, lying down, possibly standing

This self-treatment:

- relieves the squamous suture of agglutination and tension;
- relaxes the base of the skull;
- relaxes the tentorium cerebelli (the "tent of the cerebellum": an extension of the dura mater that separates the cerebellum from the lower portion of the occipital lobes);
- widens vascular passageways at the base of the skull which support the outflow of blood;
- assists in the function of some cerebral nerves, especially the vestibulo-cochlear nerve (VIII) and the vagus nerve (X);
- supports unrestricted temporal bones that mobilize the neighboring sphenoid bone and the occipital bone;
- relaxes the temporomandibular joint;
- indirectly relaxes the hyoid and the area of the throat/neck.

Performing the exercise

You relax the temporal bones through an even, very light and hardly noticeable earpull on both sides of your head.

1. Place your index fingers in the lower third of your auricles (outer ears). Your thumbs hold the auricles from behind, not touching the earlobes but clearly and firmly touching the lower part of your auricles. Preferably, let the lower jaw drop slightly. Close your eyes and feel inside.

2. With the lightness of a butterfly's wing flap, begin to pull slowly with a gentle, almost-imagined sideways tug, as even as possible and in such a way that you do not feel this as a firm pull.

    Here, too, very light but steady pulling (about 1 to 3 minutes) is preferable to fast and too much pulling! Too much sideways pulling without listening to the structures in a sensitive way can stimulate them too much. We do it just the other way round: with a gentle but continuous invitation in the direction of release, which is slightly sideways, backward and downward. Allow the structure some time, letting it decide when, where and how much tension it wants to release.

Listen to your inner doctor, telling you when your body is willing to let go and what it is willing to let go of and correct from within by itself, through your gentle invitation. Instead of forcing the structure with technical procedures, you are clear in your intention but you let the body work with its self-regulation. Listen in a relaxed way and mindfully feel what is changing, where and how.

> If the two temporal bones or the gentle pull feel different, make sure your light sideways pull is really even. It is possible that one temporal bone is less restricted than the other one. The petrous bone (Pars petrosus), a central part of the temporal bone, secures the tentorium cerebelli, which can display differing sloping and tension tendencies that can be palpated with increasing release in the area of the bones. It is fascinating to notice in the fingers and in the head that the two temporal bones are not really separate but connected via the tentorium cerebelli.

3. Slowly release the gentle earpull to the side once again. Sense how it feels now. Again palpate the craniosacral rhythm on the parietal bones (with the finger position of the previous exercise, see page 108: Has it changed, are its slow tidal movements on the left and on the right more balanced, stronger or wider?

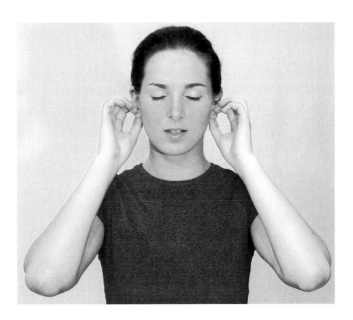

Standing: relaxing temporal bones
with gentle earpull

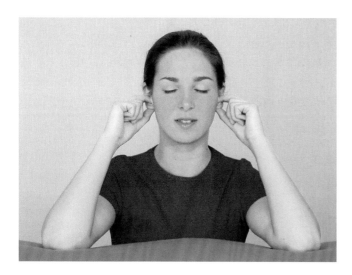

Sitting, elbows propped up:
relaxing temporal bones
with gentle earpull

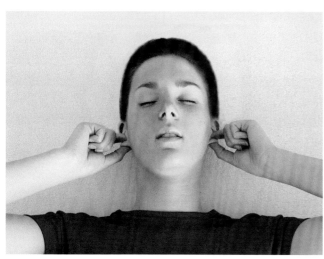

Lying down: relaxing
temporal bones
with gentle earpull

Relaxing the occipital bone (Os occipitale)   ca. 3 – 5 min.

lying down, sitting

Performing the exercise

You have already learned about various hand and finger positions for palpating the craniosacral rhythm on the occipital bone, in the exercises on pages 93, 95 and 100, with photos. There you will find information on the benefits of this self-treatment.

The lambdoid suture, which runs laterally on the occipital bone, is not to be restricted or compressed. Choose the most comfortable position on the occipital bone. This is how you can best feel the craniosacral rhythm:

- one hand across underneath or on the occipital bone, or
- both hands across, with fingers interlacing underneath or on the back of the head (the surfaces of the fingers palpate the craniosacral rhythm), or
- one hand across the upper neck area, the other hand across underneath or on the occipital bone.

Continue as previously described, points 1 to 5 on pages 106–107.

Palpating the craniosacral rhythm jointly on the frontal bone and the occipital bone:

For this you place one hand across underneath or on the occipital bone; the other one melts with much surface contact into the form of the frontal bone, without restricting any sutures.

Relaxing the nasal bone ca. 2 min.

lying down, sitting

An enjoyable relaxation exercise, particularly beneficial for people wearing glasses!

This self-treatment promotes:
- relaxation of the facial bones;
- more space for the ethmoid bone, the sense of smell;
- the flexibility of the Falx cerebri and other intracranial membranes;
- the craniosacral rhythm of the facial bones, the ethmoid bone and the sphenoid bone;
- the activity of the glands in the area of the paranasal and ethmoid sinuses, and prevents inflammations (Sinusitis maxillaris, -ethmoidalis).

Performing the exercise
1. The middle and ring finger of one hand feel the eye socket without touching the eyeballs while doing so. Both phalanxes clearly contact the upper eye sockets, at the lower part of the frontal bone, and connect with them.
2. Thumb and index finger of the other hand touch the sides of the nasal bone and connect with it. Allow yourself time until all fingertips are really connected with the touched spots. The better the connection, the easier it is for the nasal bone and the frontal nasal suture to relax.

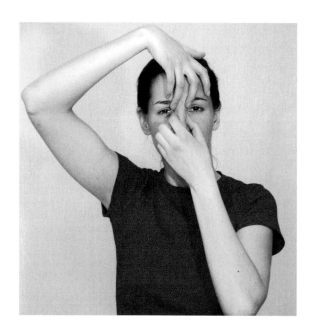

Relaxing frontal-nasal suture

3. The middle and ring finger on the eye sockets can now lightly hook into the touched surface in order not to slip off in the direction of release. If the position feels right, close your eyes and sense inside.

4. With both hands simultaneously, slowly perform a light, nearly-imagined decompression, the hands *moving away from each other*. The fingertips of the middle and ring finger, lightly hooked into the eye sockets, lightly relax the frontal bone cranially, while the thumb and index finger on the nasal bone relax it lightly, half-diagonally downward towards the floor, forward and down. The intention here is the same as in "Relaxing the temporal bones with a gentle earpull" (see pages 114–116).

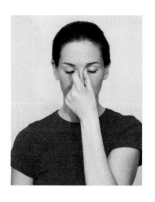

Relaxing this suture with both hands is very effective; it takes a bit of time, however, to get used to the finger position. Alternatively you can touch with index finger and thumb of one hand. The fingers are so positioned that they touch the uppermost end of the nasal bone and at the same time with their upper edge touch the eye sockets, or rather, the frontal bone. If your fingers are well connected with the level of the bones, the direction of release is away from the suture – i.e., forward (when sitting) or upward (when lying).

Feeling and relaxing the facial bones   ca. 2 – 5 min. per position

lying down, sitting

In the area of the face we are naturally particularly sensitive and we react strongly to gentle touch. When structures of the facial bones release, this also mobilizes the other cranial bones. Our senses of vision and smell also profit from this.

Compressions of the facial bones – e.g., through a collision or fall – transfer to the sphenoid bone and more or less to the entire base of the skull. A compressed or heavily agglutinated zygomatic bone influences the movements of the temporal bone – for instance, via the zygomatic arch.

This self-treatment promotes:

- relaxation of the facial bones and the previously-named structures;
- relaxation of numerous muscles, ligaments, fascia in the area of the face;
- a less restricted, more balanced craniosacral rhythm.

The photos and illustrations on pages 102–103 assist you in differentiating between the individual facial bones and subsequently finding them more easily for accurate palpation.

Performing the exercise

You touch the facial bones with several fingertips and then invite spaciousness and expanse. Whether you are sitting or lying down, the heels of the hands can touch, holding and stabilizing.

1. Loosen your arms, wrists, hands and fingers. As a greeting you slowly and lightly start touching the entire lateral area of the face and cheeks with the whole surface of your fingers. Feel the form and texture, the tonus and potential differences left and right. The surfaces of your fingers make clear contact *with the level of the bones* via skin and subcutaneous tissue. What do you perceive here? Again invite spaciousness and expanse and listen, relaxed, to the sensations. After a while remove your fingers again. How does this feel in comparison to before?

    This self-treatment can be combined with "Relaxing the eye segment," page 56.

2. Now slowly feel with your fingertips individual or various facial bones. The flexible knuckles can facilitate easy touch. When your fingertips have created clear contact with the individual facial bones, again invite spaciousness and expanse and allow the structure enough time to release. The thumbs are not involved and can lightly touch the lower jaw.

3. Occasionally the surfaces of your fingers can be positioned more to the middle or sideways towards the ears, in order to get to know, touch and relax the entire facial area.

Your fingertips touch individually, for example, the following facial bones:

Zygomatic bones and upper jaw/maxilla:
    Position 1: Ring, middle and index fingers touch the zygomatic bones, the little fingers contact the upper jaw/maxilla (right photo).
    Position 2: Middle and index fingers touch the zygomatic bones, little fingers contact the upper jaw/maxilla above the root of the nose, ring finger to the side of the nose (left photo).

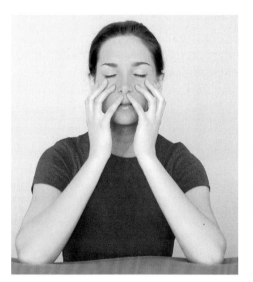
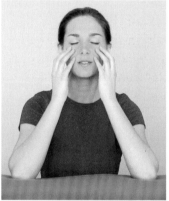

Elbows propped up: feeling and relaxing facial bones

Zygomatic bones, upper jaw/maxilla and zygomatic arch:
    Ring and middle fingers touch the zygomatic bones, index fingers touch the zygomatic arch, and little fingers contact the upper jaw/maxilla under the root of the nose or to the side of the nose.

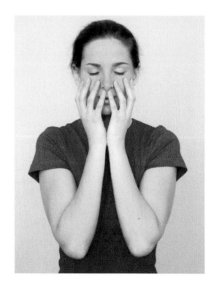

Feeling and relaxing facial bones

Relaxing the temporomandibular joints ca. 2 – 5 min.

sitting, lying down, standing

As already mentioned in the exercise "Palpating, smoothing and massaging the chewing muscles" (see page 38), our chewing musculature is often very tense and attests to the stress of our everyday life, for example through frequent clenching or nightly grinding of the teeth. Chronic tension of the muscles, ligaments, sinews and fascia around the jaw joints can overstrain these complex joints and wear them down early (one- or two-sided).

Performing the exercise

We gently touch the structures on and around the temporomandibular joint with the surfaces of our fingers. The temporomandibular joint relaxes and is relieved.

1. Place the surfaces of the index, middle and ring fingers on the side of the head, directly in front of your ears. The fingertips are positioned above the auditory canal, see right photo below. Release the lower jaw and breathe all tension felt here out through the slightly-opened mouth. Close your eyes and feel inside.

2. Via the level of the skin, the surfaces of the fingers connect with the layers of tissue, muscle and fascia underneath that are found around and above the temporomandibular joint:
   - How do they feel?
   - Do the left and right jaw joint feel different? If so, how?

3. Lighten your touch a bit without losing the clear contact with the touched structure. Do you feel warmth, expansion, the tissue getting softer? Again your touch invites spaciousness and expanse. Listen to the releases and what you thereby perceive in your body.

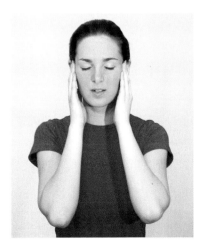 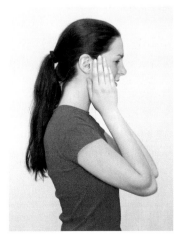

Touching and releasing tissue around jaw joints

Massage of the chewing muscles

When relaxing the facial bones and jaw joints, as well as when releasing the upper and lower jaws, the chewing muscles are also being addressed, among others. At this point be reminded of the self-massages, "Palpating, smoothing and massaging the chewing muscles" (page 38). A hearty yawn and the exercise "Stretching the face" (see page 40) can also have a releasing and regulating effect on the tonus of all chewing muscles as well as on the temporomandibular joint.

Relaxing the masseter from inside: It is possible to touch the masseter muscle from the inside (intraorally). Before you start, wash your hands well.

Performing the exercise

Open your mouth only as far as necessary to slowly and gently feel the masseter with index or little finger in the area of the cheeks from the inside. If you are not sure whether you are touching the right place, open the mouth a bit wider so that the masseter as the strongest biting, chewing muscle stretches and unmistakably reveals itself. Touch it with fingertips as soft as butter. The index or little finger is outside the row of teeth and can touch the corner of the mouth, and the mouth can be slightly closed again. Through this the masseter becomes softer and more receptive to gentle touch. While doing this breathe out all felt tensions through the slightly-open mouth.

Touching and relaxing
the upper jaw/maxilla   ca. 3 min. per position

lying down, sitting

The upper jaw bone (maxilla) consists – simplified – of two parts that are connected with each other through the median palatine suture (Sutura palatina mediana). It is linked with the sphenoid bone via the palatine bone, the vomer and the ethmoid bone. The upper jaw participates in creating the nasal cavities and sides, the hard palate and even the eye sockets. It is also important for speech and for the development of the voice. The correct bite (occlusion) is largely dependent upon a harmonious co-operation of upper and lower jaw, temporal bones, temporomandibular joint and chewing muscles.

This self-treatment promotes:
- relaxation and spaciousness for the upper jaw, and in connection with that for the palatine bone (Os palatinum), the sphenoid bone, the nasal and lacrimal bones, the ethmoid bone;
- a less restricted, more balanced craniosacral rhythm.

Find more about this in the exercise "Relaxing the nasal bone," page 117.

In the exercise "Feeling and relaxing facial bones" (page 120 or 123), the upper jaw was contacted jointly with other facial bones. Below is a specific self-treatment for the upper jaw.

Performing the exercise

First the upper jaw is touched with much surface from the outside and gently relaxed through inviting spaciousness and expansion. Afterwards the upper jaw can be relaxed with the "thumb on palate" position, by a gentle, nearly-imagined decompression.

Touching the upper jaw

Place your fingertips clearly above the upper teeth (from the outside) on the upper jaw – i.e., the little fingers underneath the root of the nose, the ring fingers closely underneath the ala of the nose (the membrane to the outside of each nostril), right next to them the middle and index fingers (tips), underneath the zygomatic arch. The thumbs are not involved or they gently touch the lower jaw.

The rest of the procedure is the same as in the exercise "Feeling and relaxing facial bones" (page121). Your fingertips slowly connect through the skin with the bone level of the upper jaw, invite spaciousness and expansion and listen to the movements and sensations.

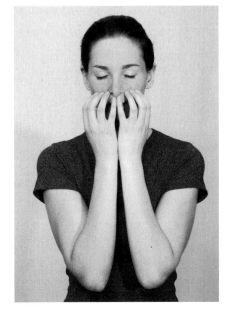

Touching the upper jaw

Relaxing the upper jaw

1. Before starting, wash your hands. "Thumb to palate" position: let your lower jaw drop and slightly open your mouth. Now slowly move your thumb (intraorally) to the middle line of the upper jaw, into the front area of the hard palate.

   On the outside, the middle phalanx of your index finger touches clearly with much surface directly under the root of the nose, above the teeth, and connects via the tissue with the upper jaw. The intensity of the touch can lighten further, the contact with the structure become even clearer.

   Note: Your lower jaw can drop in a relaxed way, the breath can flow freely. Meanwhile, consciously sense into your pelvis, ground and center yourself. You may close your eyes. Feel inside.

2. When you have an enjoyable and clear contact, **very slowly** perform a light, nearly-imagined gentle decompression; it happens steadily and more or less in the direction of the tip of the nose/chin, towards the front and down.

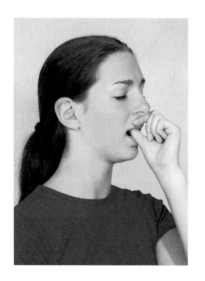 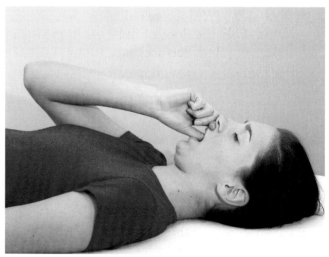

Gently relaxing upper jaw with light decompression

You do not exercise any pull; the invitation is fully sufficient! We are talking here about a hardly-noticeable decompression in which the affected structures are not over-stimulated but respected within their boundaries. During this decompression you palpate in whichever direction the varied structures relax by themselves through your invitation.

The upper jaw can relieve itself of agglutinations and compressions in various directions: away from the face towards the front, towards the feet, more towards the left or the right (as it loosens up better in one direction than the other), or in a combination of described release directions. This is why you should listen without pull as to the direction in which your upper jaw wants to release. Allow the structure enough time to harmonize itself on its own.

Relaxing the lower jaw / mandibula   ca. 2 – 5 min.

lying down, sitting

The position of this self-treatment is similar to the "Massage of the chewing muscles" (page 38) and can be combined with it. Some ideas and reasons for the relaxation of the area of lower-upper jaw/temporomandibular joint have already been shared in connection with previous exercises.

This self-treatment supports and promotes:
- releasing the temporomandibular joint, the chewing muscles, the base of the skull, the floor of the mouth, the hyoid and neck segments as well as the shoulder/neck area;
- the entire torso including pelvis and hips.

Performing the exercise

You touch the lower jaw on both sides with as much surface of your fingers as possible and continuously relax it with a gentle, nearly-imagined decompression (at an angle of about 30 to 45 degrees towards the front and downwards).

1. Extensively and comprehensively touch your lower jaw with the surfaces of your fingers: the upper part close to the jaw joints, from there the corner and the entire lower main part in the direction of the chin (see page 127, first photo).

   For this, initially place your middle and ring fingers, which are touching, with their surfaces on all these parts. The little fingers contact the ring fingers and a part of the facial muscles. The index fingers feel for the lower edge of the lower jaw and are positioned on or below this edge. Both heels of the hands or the wrists can touch and form a stabilizing pivot. Your middle, ring and index fingers connect as comprehensively as possible with the entire bony structure of the lower jaw.

Having clear contact with the level of the bones is important, as the following decompression would otherwise relax skin and connective tissue only. You may slightly increase the quality of touch in order to connect via the level of the skin, tissue, muscles, tendons and ligaments with the level of the bones. Then listen for a few moments to what the touch feels like and whether anything changes at this place and in the body in general. You might close your eyes in order to become aware of more "inside."

2. Once you have established clear contact with the area of the bony lower jaw, perform slowly and lightly a very gentle decompression: it happens steadily, more or less in direction of the chin at an angle of 30 to 45 degrees half-diagonally towards the floor (when sitting), half-diagonally towards the feet (when lying).

   For the decompression, the same goes as before with the upper jaw: the affected structures are not being stimulated through a strong, noticeable pull but are gently invited to let go of tension with the release direction of about 30 to 45 degrees. You palpate here to learn in which direction the structures want to relax.

   The lower jaw can relax in the same direction as the upper jaw: away from the face towards the front, towards the feet, sideways (left or right) and/or a combination of these. Listen to find out in which direction the lower jaw starts releasing and notice every stop when the tissue needs a break. You do not interfere with the natural self-regulation but enable it through your gentle and inviting touch.

3. During the steady decompression it is possible that the surfaces of your fingers will slide slowly and without intention slightly towards the point of the chin (as can be seen in the second photo on page 127). Despite this, stay in contact with the level of the bones of the lower jaw. Should your fingers slide even further towards the chin, release the touch. Decide whether you want to repeat the same release technique with newly-positioned fingers or whether you prefer to immediately sense into how the relaxation feels up to now.

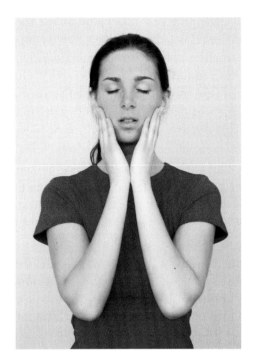
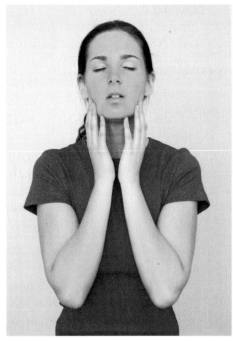
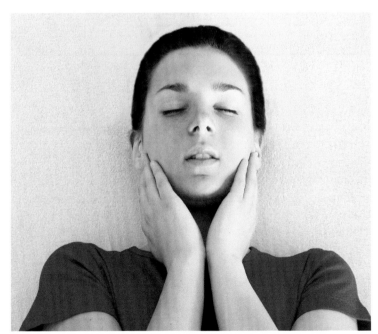

Touching and relaxing
the lower jaw

V-spread technique

ca. 2 min. per position

sitting, lying down, standing

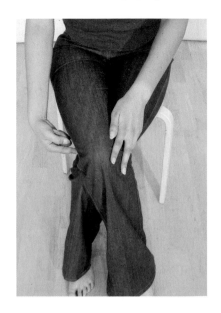

Sutherland spoke about "directing the tide." The so-called V-spread technique is an element of the treatment that focuses on directing the energy. This is easy and often very efficient. You perform this technique on the energetic level where it makes its initial impact but it goes on to affect the physical structural level. The statement "Energy follows intention" is in line with the V-spread technique where the intention is able to change the energy.

The V-spread technique offers a very gentle relaxation possibility for structures that hold fast. It can also be used to harmonize traumatized tissue, for example when you have bumped against something. The photo shows this treatment on the kneecap. V-spreading can be used all over the body, in particular on the cranial sutures.

Performing the exercise

1. Index and middle finger on one hand form a "V" and are placed with their surfaces on the structure to be balanced, in such a way that this structure is positioned between the fingers (photo: inside of the knee). The stretched index finger of the other hand touches with the fingertip opposite the "V" (photo: outside of the knee).

2. The index finger pointed towards the "V" serves as the energy-directing finger; the zone between the "V" is the place where the tension of the tissue can discharge and leave. With the energy-directing index finger you send releasing and relaxing energy to the "V." It will flow mostly diametrically through the tissue and begin releasing the tissue as well as the V-spread area. While doing this, you might visualize how the relaxing energy moves from the index finger to the holding side, then back to the index finger and from there again to the held (or traumatized) side where the energy can release in the "V" area. The structure in and around this area has the possibility of arranging itself anew.

While you are using this technique, occasionally close your eyes in order to perceive from the inside. When the relaxing effect is noticeable and enjoyable, you can apply the V-spread for about 2 to 5 minutes per position. Do you feel a difference afterwards as compared to before?

Appendix

About craniosacral therapy/ treatment

Originating in cranial osteopathy, craniosacral therapy has within the last few decades established itself and developed further as an independent therapy form. More and more physiotherapists, massage therapists, alternative practitioners, midwives and other professionals are now skilled in craniosacral therapy. It is applied in a variety of settings – for example, in rehabilitation, in care for the sick and the elderly, and in terminal care. The treatment supports babies, children and adults in their phases of growth, transformation and regeneration. Craniosacral treatment predominantly refers to the system, rather than to the symptoms. This means that by balancing the craniosacral system the body's self-healing powers are boosted and subsequently physical blockages are lessened or dissolved. Ideally you will, in addition to doing self-treatments, experience craniosacral treatments with a professional craniosacral practitioner.

Craniosacral therapy can be helpful with, for example:

- asthma
- breathing problems
- slipped disk, sciatica
- high blood pressure
- depression
- conditions of exhaustion
- hormonal dysfunctions
- hearing problems (e.g., tinnitus)
- hyperactivity
- problems with concentration and learning
- headaches, migraine
- motor and sensory dysfunctions
- sleeping disorders
- muscle spasms
- stress
- congestion problems
- problems with teeth and jaw, teeth grinding
- during and after pregnancy
- after shocks, accidents

What does a treatment with a professional craniosacral practitioner look like?

Wearing everyday clothes the client lies on a soft massage table where it is possible to relax for about an hour. The order of the treatment can vary a great deal, depending on the experience of the craniosacral practitioner, the intention of the treatment, the reaction of the client and the individual process of the session. The practitioner simply softly palpates, for example, feet, sacrum, structures on the torso, on the base of the skull and on the head (cranium). On the head the practitioner lightly touches and attends with pressure of only about 1 to 2 grams, 5 grams maximum (tiny fractions of an ounce of pressure).

The craniosacral rhythm and even slower body rhythms can often reveal themselves more freely during a craniosacral treatment. Internally, the meninges of the brain and spinal cord – the covers of our central nervous system – can be relieved of tensions, agglutinations and contortions. This process is sometimes accompanied by memories – for example, of falls, accidents or other traumatic occurrences. The temporary activation of the nervous system and the trusting attention of the therapist can help with releasing the so-called cell memory. The therapist provides space and time for this, accompanying the client and offering resources.

By being present, listening to the craniosacral rhythm and softly touching the different body parts, the practitioner supports the harmonization of the client's craniosacral system. Craniosacral practitioners primarily observe the level of the liquids, in particular the flow of the cerebrospinal fluid (Liquor cerebrospinalis). They have differing treatment approaches: biomechanical, functional or biodynamic. Interactive process monitoring as well as interlocution skills are important elements of the treatment.

A craniosacral treatment helps the body to release and relax from the outside in. At the same time various rhythms move all body structures from the inside out. These vitalizing and reorganizing movements from the center to the periphery of the body help subtly to relieve it of blockages from the midline outward. Thus the effects of a session are varied and boost healing in the body.

The professional craniosacral treatment helps harmonize various body systems in depth. This boosts the self-regulation, the self-healing powers, the strengthening of the immune system, and thus supports healing and preserving of health.

Effective non-structural elements of craniosacral treatment

This treatment has a relaxing and balancing effect, not only on the physical level. In the course of one or more craniosacral sessions you will increasingly have moments/periods where you perceive body, mind and soul no longer as separate but as a unity. If we experience, for example, spaciousness, a primal ocean of trust, peace and bliss while in deep relaxation, these are helpful resources with which we can connect increasingly in our everyday life. All these are natural core experiences when we trust and engage with them.

It appears as if in the non-structural scope of treatment it is primarily a superior natural healing principle that works for us. Perhaps it is especially the gentle, non-invasive and non-manipulative nature of craniosacral treatment that does not impede the elemental striving of nature for healing and wholeness but supports this down to the cellular level. With *craniosacral_flow*® and other gentle forms of craniosacral therapy there is hardly any manually invasive influence or pressure from the outside affecting the structure of the body. Soft touch facilitates listening to the slow rhythmic movements. Thus the skilled practitioner receives information on unrestricted as well as strained, or rather, compacted or blocked tissues that are palpated and gently released.

Physical and emotional restrictions are often linked. They are accepted and perceived, not "treated away" or broken through. Everything, even a strong tension in body structures, tells something about the story of the person. Craniosacral practitioners trust the "knowing field" and their intuition as much as the messages of the body – i.e., "the inner doctor," "the inner healer" or "the inner shaman" in the client.

Every mindful and conscious touch trains us further in listening to the healing, boosting dynamic of the body rhythms. Sensitive awareness deepens with every treatment, as much in the client as in the practitioner. This experience is never finished; it can be expanded further and it accompanies craniosacral practitioners throughout their lives.

Terms and definitions

amygdaloid body	Corpus amygdaloideum (part of the limbic system)
anatomy	science dealing with the structure of the body
anterior	forward; towards the front
arachnoid granulations	Granulationes arachnoideales; small protrusions of the arachnoid through the dura into the venous sinuses, transferring the cranial cerebrospinal fluid into the venous sinuses (so it can enter the blood stream)
arachnoid mater	Arachnoidea (mater); spiderweb-like layer of the meninges between the dura and pia mater
atlanto-occipital joint	connection of atlas and occipital bone
atlas bone	1st cervical vertebra
autonomic nervous system	part of the nervous system that is not subordinated to the influence of will and consciousness (the whole of the nerves and ganglion cells)
bregma	meeting point of sagittal and coronal sutures
caudal	downward; towards the feet (opposite of cranial)
cell memory	memory of experiences that are stored in body cells
cerebrospinal fluid	Liquor cerebrospinalis; the liquid of the brain and spinal cord
cervical vertebrae	spine in the neck area; the first seven vertebrae C1-7
chewing muscles	M. masseter; M. pterygoideus; M. temporalis
choroid plexus	Plexus choroideus; arterial node in the ventricle that produces fresh cerebrospinal fluid
coccyx	tailbone; Os coccygis
connective tissue	tissue that separates, connects, divides, covers and protects; it can be firm, elastic, like a network, or loose
contraindication	sign or reason for not using a remedy or diagnostic /therapeutic procedure
coronal suture	Sutura coronalis; connects frontal and parietal bones
coronoid process	Processus coronoideus; part of the lower jaw
cranial	of or towards the head (opposite of caudal)

cranial dura mater	Dura mater cranialis; strong connective tissue covering the brain and the inside of the skull
craniosacral rhythm	about 6 to12 cycles per minute
cranium	skull
decompression	relief of pressure
diametric	pertaining to a diameter
diaphragm	Diaphragma thora coabdominale; main breathing muscle; separates/connects chest and abdomen
drain	discharge accumulated fluid
dysfunction	malfunctioning; disorder
endocrine system	glandular system
ethmoid bone	Os ethmoidale; sieve-like bone between the eyes / eyeballs, forming the top of the inside of the upper nose
extension	opposite of flexion (see description p. 68); stretching
facial bones	viscerocranium; bones of the face
Falx cerebelli	sickle-shaped part of the dura mater, dividing the two halves of the cerebrum andconnecting the tentorium with the Foramen magnum
Falx cerebri	sickle-shaped part of the dura mater, separating the two halves of the neocortex and connecting the back and the front of the skull
flexion	opposite of extension (see description p. 56); bending
Foramen magnum	opening in the occiput for the medulla of the spine; largest opening at the base of the skull
frontal bone	Os frontale
frontonasal suture	Sutura frontonasalis; suture between the frontal and nasal bones
fulcrum	point on which something turns or pivots
hyoid bone	Os hyoideum; supports the muscles of the tongue
hypophysis	pituitary gland resting in the sphenoid bone
iliac bone	Crista iliaca; one of the three bones of the innominate or hip bone
iliosacral joint	joint connecting sacrum and iliac bones
indication	reason for applying a specific diagnostic or therapeutic procedure
intraorally	inside the mouth
ischium	Os ischii; either of the bones on which the body rests when sitting

lateral	side; sideways; to the side
ligament	band of tissue connecting two bones/structures with each other or holding an organ in place
long-tide	tidal movement with about 1 cycle per 100 seconds
lumbar spine	the 5 vertebrae in the lower back
lumbosacral joint	L5/S1; connection of the lowest lumbar vertebra with the sacrum
major (greater) trochanter	bony protrusion near the end of the femur (thigh bone)
mandible	inferior maxillary bone; lower jaw bone
mastoid process	processus mastoideus; bony prominence of the temporal bone behind and below the ear
maxillary bone	upper jaw; Os maxillare
medial	towards the middle
meninges	membranes covering the brain and spinal cord
mid-tide	tidal movement with about 2 to 3 cycles per minute
mobility	overall flexibility; ability to reposition
motility	individual flexibility within; intrinsic movement; ability to move spontaneously
motor neuron	nerve cell that transmits muscle impulses
nasal bone	Os nasale
occipital bone	Os occipitale; occiput
occipital condyle	Condylus occipitalis; cranial part of the atlanto-occipital joint; protrusions on the back of the skull which connect with the atlas vertebra
occlusion	the way the teeth fit together when biting
OIR	outer-inner rotation, as in flexion/extension
palatine bone	Os palatinum; bone at the roof of the mouth
palpate	feel for, sense (perceive and distinguish through touching and feeling)
parietal bone	Os parietale; bone covering the top of the head
pathological	sick; signifying an illness or pathology
peristalsis	digestive movements and noises of stomach and intestines
petrous bone	Pars petrosus; part of the temporal bone
pia mater	soft part of the meninges directly adhering to the brain and spinal cord
pineal gland	Corpus pineale; epiphysis

posterior	backward, towards the rear
PRM	primary respiratory mechanism
receptors	nerve cells for perceiving particular stimuli
rectus abdominis muscle	Musculus rectus abdominis; major abdominal muscle connecting pubic bone and sternum
regulation	arrangement of the organ systems of a living organism through various control devices (e.g. hormones, nerves); automatic adjustment of a living being to changing environmental conditions by maintaining a physiological condition of balance
resorb	take in (e.g., dissolved substances into the bloodstream); re-absorb
rhythm	evenly-structured movement; periodic change; regular repetition of natural processes
sacrum	Os sacrum
sagittal suture	Sutura sagittalis
scope, spectrum	amplitude (of the craniosacral rhythm)
self-palpation	feeling/sensing your body with your fingers/hands
solar plexus	autonomic nerve plexus for the upper abdomen
sphenoid bone	Os sphenoidale; at the base of the skull, behind the eyes
spinal dura mater	Dura mater spinalis, dural tube
spine	Columna vertebralis
squamous suture	Sutura squamosa
statics	bodies at rest or in equilibrium; in natural balance
sternum	breastbone
stillpoint	healing pause in the cranial rhythm or slower rhythms
sutures	differently-formed seams or connections between bones
symptom	sign of a particular illness; characteristic pathological change belonging to a particular disease pattern
temporal bone	Os temporale
temporal muscle	Musculus temporalis
thalamus	part of the diencephalon of the brain; collection and changeover point for inner and outer stimuli; gateway to the consciousness
therapeutic pulse	physical energetic indication of release of tension in the tissue

thoracic inlet	Apertura thoracica; upper opening of the chest cavity
thoracic vertebrae 1 – 12	the 12 vertebrae which are connected to ribs on each side
thymus gland	gland above the heart and behind the sternum; primary organ of the lymphatic system; produces T-lymphocytes important for immunization
tonus	condition of slight tension (partial contraction) in muscle tissue
vagus nerve	Nervus vagus; cranial nerve X; longest nerve of the parasympathetic nervous system
venous sinus	Sinus venosus; large cavity in the cranium; cerebrospinal fluid flows through the arachnoid granulations into the venous sinuses and thence into the veins/bloodstream
visceral	referring to the inner organs or viscera
visualize	imagine something visually
vomer	Os vomer; plow-shaped bone, part of the septum inside the nose
V-spread technique	energy-directing technique
zygomatic bone	Os zygomaticum

Bibliography

Agustoni, D. *Craniosacral Rhythm: A practical guide to a gentle form of bodywork therapy*. Churchill Livingstone/Elsevier, ISBN 978-0443-067372

Becker, R.E. *The Stillness of Life*. Stillness Press, ISBN 978-0-9675851-1-6

Calais-Germain, B. *Anatomy of Movement*. Eastland Press, ISBN 978-0-939616-17-6

Chaitow, L. *Palpation and Assessment Skills*. Churchill Livingstone, ISBN 978-0443072185

Damasio, A. *Descartes' Error: Emotion, reason and the human brain*. G.P. Putnam's Sons, ISBN 978-009950164-0

Kern, M. *Wisdom in the body*. Thorsons, ISBN 978-0-7225-3708-4

Levine, P.A. and A. Frederick. *Waking The Tiger: Healing trauma*. North Atlantic Books, ISBN 978-155643233-0

Levine, P.A. *Healing Trauma. Book and CD*, Sounds True Audio, ISBN 978-159179247-5

Liem, T. *Craniosacral Osteopathy: Principles and practice*. Elsevier, ISBN 978-0-443-07499-8

Lipton, B. *Biology of Belief*. Mountain of Love/Elite Books, ISBN 978-097599147-3

Oschman, J. *Energy Medicine: The scientific basis*. Churchill Livingstone, ISBN 978-0-443-06261-2

Pert, C.B. *Molecules of Emotion: Why you feel the way you feel*. Scribner, ISBN 978-0-684-83187-9

Heller, L., D. Pool Heller and Peter Levine. *Crash Course: A self-healing guide to auto accident trauma and recovery*. North Atlantic Books, ISBN 978-155643372-6

Ridley C. *Stillness–Biodynamic Cranial Practice and the Evolution of Consciousness*. North Atlantic Books, ISBN 978-1-55643-592-8

Shea, M.J. *Biodynamic Craniosacral Therapy*. North Atlantic Books, ISBN 978-155643591-1

Sutherland, W.G. *Teachings in the Science of Osteopathy*. Sutherland Cranial Teaching Foundation, ISBN 978-0-930298-00-5

Upledger, J.E. *Your Inner Physician and You*. North Atlantic Books, ISBN 978-155643-246-0

Upledger, J.E. and J.D. Vredevoogd. *CranioSacral Therapy*. Eastland Press, ISBN 978-0-939616-01-5

Upledger, J.E. and R. Grossinger. *SomatoEmotional Release: Deciphering the language of life*. North Atlantic Books, ISBN 978-1-55643-412-9

Recommended Music (selection)

Agustoni, Daniel / Wiese, Klaus. *Harmonizing your Craniosacral System.* Findhorn Press, ISBN 978-1-84409-126-3

Deuter, Chaitanya H.:
- *REIKI – Hands of Light.* New Earth Records, NE 9806-2
- *Wind & Mountain, Healing Music.* The Relaxation Company, CD 3183
- *Sea and Silence.* New Earth Records, CD 77159
- *Earth Blue.* New Earth Records, CD 77164

Kamal. *Reiki Whale Song.* New Earth Records, CD 77154

Naegele, David. *Temple in the Forest; Valley of the Sun.* New World, CD 105

Wiese, Klaus / Ted de Jong / M. Grassow. *El-Hadra, the Mystic Dance.* Edition AK/ Silenzio Music

Wiese, Klaus: *Mudra.* Aquamarin, CD 6294

Acknowledgements

My heartfelt gratitude is due to all those who have supported me in developing this book. Special thanks go to Petra Reinmuth who supported me in all stages of this book project and who has for years competently accompanied me to courses in Switzerland and abroad. I would also like to express my gratitude to Heini Müller and Joachim Lichtenberg for their feedback.

Thank you to Tom Schneider and Anuschka Colonnello for the photo shooting, and to Christine Mäder for actively assisting me in the office of the Sphinx Institute.

Thanks are due to Mr. Marcus Sommer and Professor Dr. Johannes Rohen for permission to use the illustration of the colored skull, and in particular to Dr. Rohen for his excellent anatomy books with their functional, holistic approach.

A big thank-you to Findhorn Press, Sabine Weeke and Jean Semrau for the very good collaboration.

Thank you to Peter Levine and the entire assisting team of the Somatic Experiencing Training II Switzerland.

I would like to express my sincere gratitude to all my teachers who have instructed me in diverse approaches of craniosacral treatment. Special thanks to Dr. William Martin Allen for his teaching at our Institute and for writing the Foreword to this book.

And of course many thanks to all my clients as well as all participants in my craniosacral training courses, who have given and still give me the opportunity to continue my learning.

Self-Treatments Combined

Possible combinations from Parts 1, 2 and 3 – three examples

Example 1
Shaking and loosening the body, p. 29
Palpating, smoothing and massaging the chewing muscles, p. 38
Sensing and observing the breath, breathing exercise "Circular breathing," p. 45
Resources: to connect yourself consciously with power sources, p. 46
Holistic body awareness, p. 59
Observing the craniosacral rhythm or slower rhythms on thighs, sides of the pelvis and head, p. 64
Perceiving and differentiating body rhythms, p. 61
Relaxing the connective tissue with light fascia gliding (1-2 positions), p. 89
Feeling and relaxing the cranial sutures (1-2 positions), p. 103
Activating the stillpoint in the occipital bone, p. 88
Gentle earpull, p. 114
Touching and relaxing the sacrum and the occipital bone, p. 82
Sensing the sacrum, the spine and their connection to the occipital bone, p. 48
Sensing feet, legs, pelvis, sacrum: grounding, centering, connecting, p. 47

Example 2
Muscle tapping, jogging and vibrating, p. 30
Stretching and straightening the body, p. 31
Relaxing the costal (rib) arch, p. 34
Belly massage, p. 36
Palpating, smoothing and massaging the chewing muscles, p. 38
Resources: to connect yourself consciously with power sources, p. 46
Sensing feet, legs, pelvis, sacrum: grounding, centering, connecting, p. 47
Sensing ribcage, shoulder blades, shoulders, arms, cervical spine, head, p. 50
Holistic body awareness, p 59
Observing the craniosacral rhythm or slower rhythms on thighs, sides of the pelvis and head, p. 64
Perceiving and differentiating body rhythms, p. 61
Activating the stillpoint in the pelvis, p. 87
Relaxing the connective tissue (2-3 positions), p. 89
Gentle earpull, p. 114
Sensing sacrum, spine and their connection to the occipital bone, p. 48
Sensing feet, legs, pelvis, sacrum: Grounding, centering, connecting, p. 47

Example 3

Tapping the thymus gland, p. 32
Scalp massage, p. 41
Ear massage, p. 42
Resources: to connect yourself consciously with power sources, p. 46
Sensing sacrum, spine and their connection to the occipital bone, p. 48
Sensing individual body parts, p. 51
Holistic body awareness, p. 59
Observing the craniosacral rhythm or slower rhythms on thighs, sides of the
    pelvis and head, p. 64
Relaxing the connective tissue (3-4 positions), p. 89
Feeling and relaxing the facial bones, p. 119
Feeling, relaxing and massaging the cranial sutures (3-4 positions), p. 103
Gentle earpull, p. 114
Relaxing the sacrum in supine position (2-3 positions), p. 74
Activating the stillpoint in the pelvis, p. 87
Sensing and observing the breath, p. 44
Sensing feet, legs, pelvis, sacrum: grounding, centering, connecting, p. 47

A – Z summary of self-treatments

Addresses and information

Information on talks, introductory training in craniosacral therapy and self-treatment with Daniel Agustoni:

Sphinx-Craniosacral-Institute
Postfach 629, CH – 4003 Basel, Switzerland
Tel +41 (0) 61 274 07 74, Fax +41 (0) 61 274 07 75
eMail: sphinx@craniosacral.ch
Homepage: www.craniosacral.ch

The author is available for craniosacral seminars worldwide. He offers introductory courses, trainings in craniosacral_flow®, advanced courses, holiday courses.

Addresses of craniosacral therapists on the Internet
    www.iahp.com
    www.ccst.co.uk
    www.craniosacral.co.uk
    www.craniosacralflow.ch
    and via various search engines

Addresses of therapists trained in Somatic-Experiencing®
    www.traumahealing.com

The colored model of the skull originates from SOMSO MODELL. Further information on the Internet: www.somso.de; eMail: somso@t-online.de

Companion CD

This CD contains 17 exercises for relaxation, awareness and self-treatment, each between 1 and 15 minutes in length:

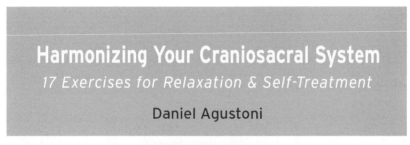
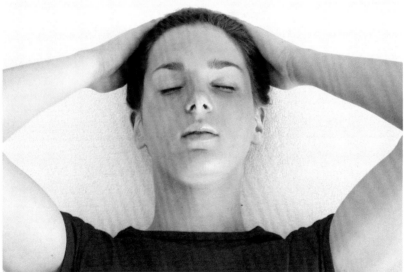

Music by Klaus Wiese, musician and sound researcher, whose CDs include *El-Hadra, Monsoon, ZEN, Soma, Touch of Silence*. Voice: Shirley Barthelmie. Duration: 69:31 minutes. ISBN 978-1-84409-126-3.

Available from your local bookstore, or directly from www.findhornpress.com

Also by Daniel Agustoni

Craniosacral Rhythm: A practical guide to a gentle form of bodywork therapy.
Churchill Livingstone/Elsevier, ISBN 978-0443-06737-2

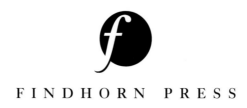

FINDHORN PRESS

Books, Card Sets,
CDs & DVDs
that inspire and uplift

For a complete catalogue,
please contact:

Findhorn Press Ltd
305a The Park, Findhorn
Forres IV36 3TE
Scotland, UK

Telephone +44-(0)1309-690582
Fax +44-(0)1309-690036
eMail info@findhornpress.com

or consult our catalogue online
(with secure order facility) on
www.findhornpress.com